RISE & SHINE

6 Master Steps to
Get Moving

PAMELA HUNTER

CCA, E-RYT, INHC
Director of Joyful Healing
Open Your Wings LLC

Rise & Shine:
6 Master Steps to Get Moving
Pamela Hunter

Illustrations by: Carole Stone Carson
CaStone Design & Art

Cover Design by: Melissa Noto Design Studios Ltd.

This book is printed in the United States of America

I dedicate this book

To my husband George, who has supported me and given me

the freedom to grow,

To my teacher, Stacey, who helped me find my authentic self,

To my boys, Ben and Charlie, who challenge and love me,

To all my teachers and students along the way who have

changed my life

(You know who you are) and

To my parents for always believing in me.

Table of Contents

1

Own It

Your Story, Your Idea, Your Knowledge, & Your Expertise

INTRODUCTION

I grew up in a dynamic, entrepreneurial family. Dad was a real motivator and a person who lived and still lives life to the fullest. He built his business from scratch and treated all those who worked with him like family. This created a swinging door to our lives so business became 'our everything'. Events, meetings, and business people crowded together in our home, creating a flow of electrified energy that kept us all going at full tilt. I loved it, thrived on it, and to this day model my own life after a father who woke me up every morning and said, "Rise and shine. Time to start a great day!"

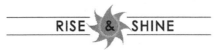

We learned very early how to take care of simple and complicated tasks; this was all taught by watching, learning, trusting, and doing. We all had responsibilities to take care of the house and our 'toys', including mini bikes, riding lawn mower, and motor home. We never knew when Dad would come home with business people or invite friends to join us for dinner. Dad not only motivated his family and his employees, but everyone he met along the way. His words still ring in my ears till this day, "Ten percent of your attitude comes from what you were given. The other 90% is what you make it to be. "

Looking back, while he taught us about responsibilities and taking care of material things, he was also teaching us life skills and trusting us to be responsible. This created a true respect and a sense of knowing in all of my family. We never questioned; we just knew. He instilled a sense of knowing inside of us by trusting us to make the right decisions for ourselves. Call it confidence, wisdom, awareness; it is all of these and so much more.

I was not a typical little kid. Being the youngest of four, I enjoyed the booming years of Dad's business all during my childhood. I could be found attending the dinner business meetings or entertaining the monthly sales team of twenty plus people we hosted at home. These were the days when children were better seen and not heard, but my dad allowed me to have a voice through my entertainment skills. I played backgammon with the sales team and often won money from them, which was put towards my college fund. They bet with the cute little girl who graciously beat them, badly!

My fondest memories of growing up were motor homing on the weekends with my family in our white Winnebago with a big green stripe that drew a big W across the side. On Friday afternoons, we would each pack a grocery bag with clothes, take our bag to the rig, remove our clothes from the bag, fold up the bag in the bottom of our drawer, and place the clothes on top. That was our space – organized and concise. We would then travel with the Motor Home Association to different parts of the country. I had a special seat on a ledge directly behind the driver, my dad. It was my responsibility to stay up with him at night and keep him awake. We had fun on the CB. My dad's handle was Greenhead (a big hunter of Mallard ducks) and I was Motor Mouth Mama coming at ya!

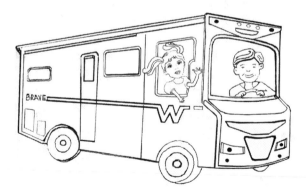

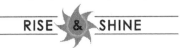
I considered this my sacred, quiet time with Dad. The dark roads were lit with only the headlights and taillights of other cars. The moon and the stars shone brightly on some nights and on others not at all. He shared his early life of having grown up on a farm in Southern Illinois. Dad's stories were rich with life lessons because he came from so little and developed it into so much!

Dad played baseball in high school and began dating my mom when he was thirteen years old! He and his brothers were boys of those times, going to school, working in the fields, and using their spare time to enjoy cars and girls. One day, his brother found their dad's clippers and instead of waiting on their dad to cut their hair, they all began cutting each other's in the flat top style. This inspired my dad to go away to barber college at age eighteen but not for long. He was in love with my mom and heartbroken by the distance, so he quit college and came home to cut hair to be with her. Working in the barbershop, he cut thirty-two heads a day!

The barbershop shared space with IBM. Everyday my dad would hear the IBM guys tell each other their stories of glory and wealth and how they only worked three days a week. This was inspiring, but he often wondered how well they would do if they worked a full week. Insurance agents came in for their bi-weekly trims and talked a lot about their success stories. Dad knew with his attitude of working the 90% of what you can control would serve him well if he could get hired at IBM; unfortunately at the time, they would not give him an interview without a college degree. However, the insurance guys heard his motivating attitude and hired him straight away. He cut hair during the day and sold insurance at night. He quickly became their top insurance sales person!

Dad knew Sales was in his blood, so he went into sales full time with 3M selling copy machines. The rest is history; he found a business partner, moved to Jefferson City, Missouri (where I was raised) and began growing his company, Modern Business Systems. He was living his dream, building relationships, motivating others, and growing a family.

Dad always added at the conclusion of his story that all of this would not have been possible if it hadn't been for the love of his life, a thirteen-year-old girl, who would later become his bride. He really believed behind every great man is an even greater woman.

Modeling this success I witnessed through my mom and dad, I found life to move along easily and was abundant with many accomplishments. I didn't realize it at the time, but I took most everything I did as serious as a grown up would take a career. And with this way of thinking, I became an all or nothing type personality. I gave it my all, or not at all. I know this sounds like perfectionism? This personality trait served me well in my early days with many awards and accomplishments. I was a big fish in a little pond with tons of

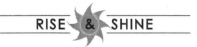

support all around me. One of my biggest accomplishments in high school was creating a PEER Counseling program for our school of approximately 2800 peers. My junior and senior year was all about helping others with drug addiction, teen pregnancy, divorce, self-esteem, and much more. These efforts gifted me the American Legion Award upon graduation.

However, I was tapped out and worn out by the end of high school and ready to move on. My sister gave me good advice when she told me to go have fun during college and to be all right with the role of a little fish in a big pond. Knowing this was great advice, that is what I did, but then I crashed! Without having a project or a passion, I found myself lost without my normal sense of devotion to voice, write, share, or live with love. This threw me into a state of depression!

After a while, depression became an intolerable way of being to me, so I set about creating the **6 Master Steps to Get Moving** and thus began my own journey of discovery, evolution, and developing myself into a whole person using Dad's simple words as an inspiration, "Rise and Shine."

MY STORY

I used to be what I call a happy depressed person. I smiled when around people even though most of the time I felt alone, especially during my early days in college when finding myself in an environment full of people who thought four years funded by Mom and Dad was an opportunity to play all day and party all night. Not me. I couldn't balance both work and play. I took everything in life seriously and wanted to accomplish something great but wasn't mature enough to know what that comprised at the time.

I knew intuitively the world had something special for me, big plans were in the works but hadn't revealed themselves to me, nor did I know how to go about realizing my higher purpose without even a hint of what that entailed. Looking back at my miserable, depressed state, I realized not knowing what the world knew was enough to depress the most joyous spirit. When scrutinizing my state of mind, I also realized part of my depression had been caused by not loving my true self and not being around people who loved me just because I am me, and not because they are under the false impression I'm somebody else.

My real self differed greatly from the other self who tended to be judgmental and was easily aggravated by the behaviors of those around me. Of course, my frustration over my surroundings not being up to par and general need for

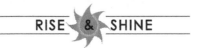

a stimulating environment caused me to become agitated, which resulted in my going about the campus feeling lost and useless.

Fortunately, I could talk openly to my family. I told them everything and even made a couple of faulty innuendoes about college might not be the right venue for all my unsung talents and me. Motivator Dad came to the rescue by forcing me to make a plan. I had heard these words throughout childhood and well, frankly, I thought I had made a plan, just not the right one for me. He gave me a serious look at my future without a college education, and no, I couldn't see myself working weekends on a retail sales floor my entire life and not having the credentials to accomplish more.

He said, "You're a woman in the 90s, and a woman has to have a college education to be able to take care of herself." He even went on to say it was expected of me in our current society. I hadn't thought of myself as having a place in society. Actually, putting myself in any social norm wasn't something that had entered my head at that time. Nonetheless, after listening to Dad's pep talk, I felt better, perked up, and put my ear to what else he had to say.

"It's time you look at college as a career that has a salary attached to it." He gave me a year's salary to pay for my expenses, tuition, and anything else I actually needed to commit fully to the idea of now viewing college as a career.

Somehow, this made the whole concept of college palatable. First, I owned the situation by going to the bank and putting a certain amount in CDs for future expenses. I even found a job selling Kirby vacuum cleaners and after only selling three, I now had an extra $1000, which allowed me some breathing room with my expenses, even though I had plenty of money.

I then chose to transfer to University of Missouri but in order to graduate I would need to have 45 credits in my own major of Fashion Merchandising and Marketing. MU wouldn't allow me to take as many hours as my own major required, so I enrolled in a college just thirty minutes away. I attended both schools simultaneously in order to meet my goal of graduating in four years. Everyone thought I was insane when taking 26 hours in one semester during my final year. I reached my goal with a high grade point average. University of Missouri applied my credit hours from the other school to my major and allowed me to graduate at my personal goal of four years.

My family took me out to dinner to celebrate and Dad raised his glass in a toast of congratulation, "Cheers to Pam. She owns graduating in four years. This is a great accomplishment!"

I felt on top of the world for years while working in my chosen profession, married to the love of my life, my best friend, and feeling like a contributing member of society and my

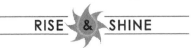
family. Then I became pregnant and was put on bed rest with preterm labor; this was enough to curtail my enthusiasm for my unilateral career goals. Not returning to work and staying home as a mom threw me back into my old depression, but this time I wasn't so far gone I didn't know enough to make another plan, which encompassed the added responsibility of now having two dependents back to back – two gorgeous little boys with the older assessed with special needs at the age of three. I needed to find a way of helping my child while helping myself maintain the equilibrium necessary to deal with life's new challenges. I truly believe we moms must help ourselves before we can help our kids.

I went to my first yoga class in 1999 on a friend's recommendation and was immediately hooked and was blissed on this new practice. After practicing yoga seriously with my teacher every day and often twice daily, I became a yogini and achieved many certifications. A whole new world opened up to me through yoga. I felt at home. While working in the yoga studio, I was introduced to many other modalities. As a YogaKids® teacher, tools came to me to help my son who was struggling with Sensory Integration, OT, PT, and Speech issues as well as asthma and allergies.

Reiki was also a technique I learned to help my son and myself relax at the end of the day or whenever needed for comfort. Essential oils were a Godsend while teaching a kids yoga class one morning. A colleague in the studio helped me out by applying a couple of oils Raven™ and RC™ to my chest and my back to help support my respiratory system, so I could breathe through my last class. Later that night, I went home to see my son struggling on all types of asthma and allergy medications. I then was educated about the power of Young Living Essential Oils and ordered them for him. After two months of applying these same two oils to his chest and back, his respiratory system became healthy. We never refilled his medications again! The holistic modalities (Reiki, cranial sacral therapy, yoga breathing, and essential oils) we used in his early years, coupled with the in-school and out-of-school therapies for OT, PT, and Speech helped him go from having personal aides in kindergarten and first grade to testing out of his IEP (Individual Education Plan) by fourth grade. He joyfully healed and support was no longer necessary. He is at present on scholarship at The Ohio State for trumpet performance. This requires him to rehearse several hours a day, so I consider it amazing he can blow a horn for that long on a consistent basis.

Ben's holistic triumph was a major turning point for our whole family. I rode along on my own enthusiasm to combine yoga with energy work and essential oils giving me certifications in all areas. I not only helped my family and myself but also began helping others.

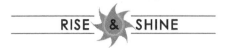
TAKING OWNERSHIP OF MY STORY

*Loving ourselves through the process of owning
our story is the bravest thing we'll ever do.*

- Brené Brown

Yoga gave me the oxygen and space needed to come into my own light and power. I discovered this practice possessed many aspects: postures, breathing, and chanting, which can also be incorporated into the practice to rebalance the nervous system. Using all three, I found an awareness that helped me work through the emotions that were stuck in my body. It also helped to strengthen my body and mind. This increased awareness within myself allowed me to heal my own depression and anxiety. Gradually, I threw out all the allopathic medicines in our cabinet and began using oils, yoga, breathing, and energy. I then began to make several life changes including learning about organic foods, introducing vegetables and greens into my diet, such as kale, collards, spinach, and the almighty beet. Blood builder beet soup became a staple. This required me to eliminate my everlasting love for my favorite comfort foods: diet coke, Dr. Pepper, Taco Bell, and periodic fast food trips to satisfy my French fry attacks. This did not happen overnight. It was a journey in itself. I still feel to this day awareness is the greatest gift yoga has given to my family and me. I take ownership of my story by living it!

TAKING OWNERSHIP OF MY IDEA

Taking ownership to combine yoga, energy work, and essential oils gave me the energy to create the Rise and Shine morning practice. Most of us know depression can creep up on us during the night so to ease the sensation of wanting to stay in bed, I developed a simplistic series of Rise and Shine movements to wake up the body from the toes to the head while rising from bed.

POINT AND FLEX

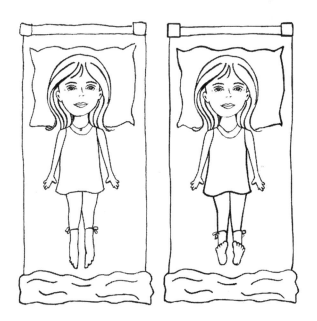

* Breathe in as you point your toes
* Breathe out as you flex your feet
* Repeat 3x

gets the Lymphatic System moving

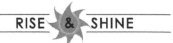
ANKLE CIRCLES

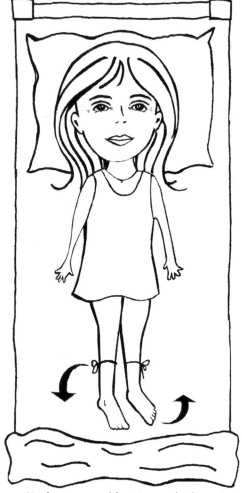

* Circle your ankles 3x each direction
* Remember to breathe
  supports circulation

SELF HUG

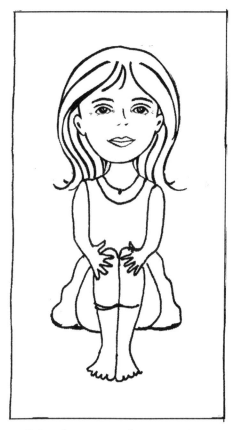

* Bring knees to chest in a hug
* Love yourself

supports digestive system

ROLLING OUT OF BED

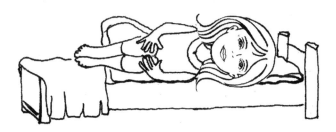

* Roll over to one side to get out of bed
* Be in fetal postion, use top hand against bed to push yourself up to seated
* Swing legs around, touch the floor

The healthy way to get out of bed

TARZAN TAP

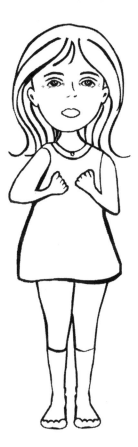

* Standing on floor, tap chest like Tarzan
* You can add sound if you want (ah-ah)

supports the immune system

EXTENDED MOUNTAIN POSE

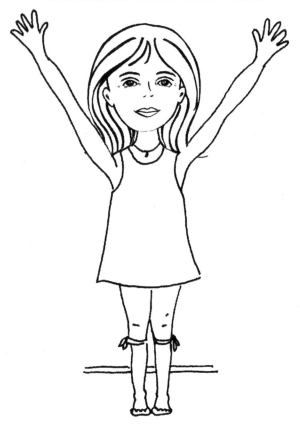

* Stand with feet parallel under your hips
* Lengthen arms up to the sky
* Breathe in and out

supports the whole body

STANDING TWISTS

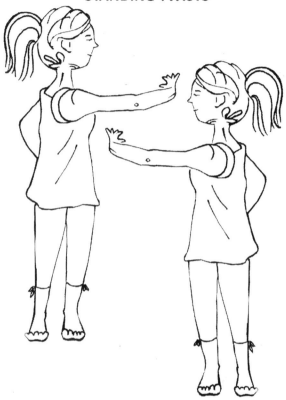

* Twisting, push the air with the hand on each side
* Inhale when twisting left
* Exhale when twisting right

blood and oxygen moving

NECK CIRCLES

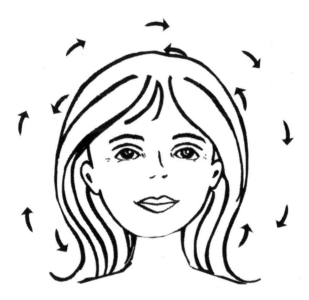

* Circle your neck slowly and gently 3x each direction
* Inhale back/ exhale forward
   If it is too much to circle all the way around, then half circles are good too
* Drop head forward and move from shoulder to shoulder

supports the nervous system

RAG DOLL

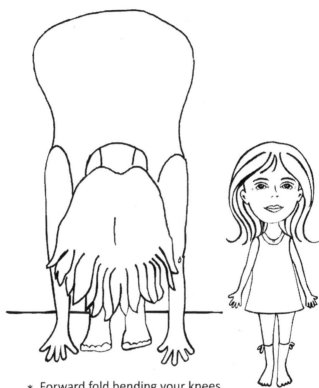

* Forward fold bending your knees
* Hang like a rag doll - let yourself relax
* To come up, place hands on lower back
* Stand up with flat back

helps let go of tension

PRAYER TO HEART

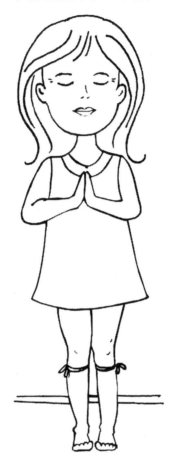

Rise and shine to a great day!

I often say to my class, "Through awareness, we transform the body and the mind to meet the soul." I really believe this and now the smile on my face comes from a place of genuine contentment.

My own teacher and best friend Stacy Vann always said, "Life is not an emergency." I thought this statement the most brilliant thing I had ever heard surpassing all existential philosophies and psychoanalytic theories. Yes, definitely, if taken to heart, 'life is not an emergency' could change a person's outlook and lift the heaviness while in the process of living. It did mine. I gave up thoughts of depression altogether and chose to live in the moment, ready to serve others by modeling the freedom I had found through self-love and awareness. I wanted to be the teacher who could meet people where they are and help them to find their path to their own freedom.

I anoint my heart with three drops of the essential oil Believe™ to stay on track with my ideas and feel faith, hope, health, happiness, and vitality. Gary's Good Day Protocol is always helpful on a daily basis by enjoying 1 to 3 drops of Valor® on my feet, Harmony™ around my navel, Joy™ on my heart, and White Angelica™ on my shoulders. This protocol supports feelings of courage, harmony, joy, and protection.

I had found my own path and now knew what the world had in mind for me. I would combine my passions and OWN all aspects of my business - yoga, essential oils, and healing work to help others and myself with wellness, purpose, and abundance, and in fact, I would call my business Joyful Healing. The sunshine not only came back into my life, I became the sun!!! I OWNED IT!!!

YOU HAVE TO OWN IT

BELLY BREATHING

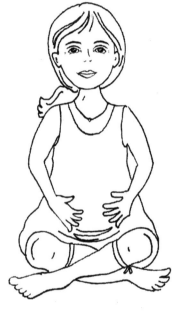

*Inhale, fill your belly like a big balloon.

*Exhale, let the belly (balloon) deflate.

SEE BREATHING APPENDIX I

No matter whether you are planning a business, a family, a fun trip, a diet plan, a workout, or a lifestyle change you have to OWN IT. In order to own my business, I had to acknowledge that I actually had something going on that deserved all the energy and attention necessary to make it work. I realized I, like other people, craved three things: energy, attention, and vitality. When I gave myself these three things, I realized who I am, what I wanted, and where I am going. I often gave my attention to everyone else and when I discovered I needed some of my own attention, it was a revelation to me. I brought energy, attention, and vitality into my life with the use of essential oils, yoga poses, and breathing practices.

Once I began to own my story and my idea, it was time to take ownership of my body of knowledge and expertise I had gained over the years. Yoga, energy work, and essential oils ceased being a hobby and became something I could share with the world, and like my father, I incorporated caring for my family and my business into my daily life. We all experienced remarkable transformations daily.

I traveled to Utah and met the owner D. Gary Young of Young Living Essential Oils. I wanted to know who and what he was about. I went with him to see the plants and oils at the source, from Seed to Seal®. We visited Utah, Idaho, France and Ecuador. I even journeyed the Frankincense trail from Egypt to Jordan. I was so blissed out on oils that I incorporated them into every part if my family's life, and mine and then into my Yoga and Healing business.

Initially, I experimented by personally using oils in every way including: inhalation, diffusing, topically, down the hatch,

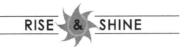

up the yoni, and an inch back where the sun doesn't shine. I have even done IV essential oils treatments after being diagnosed in 2009 with having eight fibroid tumors. Wanting to be treated naturally and without the risk of surgery, I went to the Nova Vita Clinic in Ecuador where I was given Frankincense, Balsam Fir, and Helichrysum® intravenously. Later that night, the cleansing began. Every gastronomical orifice spoke to me that night. I spent hours hugging the porcelain bowl, sitting on the porcelain bowl, and staring at the porcelain bowl waiting for my next round of purification experience. My entire body shook with releasing sensations and simultaneous relief to be rid of the toxins polluting it. (This gastronomical incident, I realized, had been made more dramatic by having eaten a New York style pizza in Miami while on layover to Ecuador.) Oddly enough with every release, I felt blessed!

The next morning, the fibroid pain had disappeared and my body sang with happiness from feeling so clean and even pure. I had no desire to put anything into my new sparkling body. Two days later, I went back to the clinic to receive another IV treatment using the Young Living Oil Thieves®. This gave me enormous energy and left me with a feeling of euphoria. I wanted to keep this feeling of high energy and purity so began to fast by only eating small portions of veg-etables for the next twelve days.

The yeast (candida) in my body dissipated, brain fog was lifted, I stopped having food cravings, lost excess weight, and miraculously the pain from the fibroids disappeared completely. When I came home, I decided to keep a clean, grain free diet, eliminating sugar and dairy (with the exception of goat cheese). I dropped thirty pounds in three months! I stuck to a regimen of fish, chicken, vegetables, red potatoes only, and a small amount of fruit. My green Vitamix® drinks with fresh veggies and rice bran protein (PowerMeal™ from Young Living) was a staple. I felt transformed. I began to live what I was to preach. I began to tell people I am a product of the product.

TAKING OWNERSHIP OF MY KNOWLEDGE AND EXPERTISE

I took ownership by sharing my expertise and knowledge with all my communities. I spoke about the twelve Biblical oils at church. I used them to anoint the children in the children's mass. I put oils in the water for the washing of the feet during Lenten services. I would do prayer services based on Frankincense, Myrrh, and Thieves®. I helped the children and their families in my neighborhood by using oils to ease the discomfort of bee stings, cuts, scrapes, bruises, burns, as well as support healthy immune systems. One day I was The Yoga Lady and the next day I became The Oil

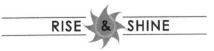

Lady. I used oils in my yoga classes to support breathing, help alleviate old trauma and other negative emotions, and help relax muscles and achy bones. I used oils on my family to support healthy respiratory functions, help relax seasonal discomforts, promote good sleep patterns, and help calm occasional headaches. In my Joyful Healing practice, I anointed clients with essential oils to support energy and wellness in all areas: physical, emotional, mental, social, and spiritual. My intention was always to bring comfort and calming peace, which I was able to do by using relaxation oils such as Peace and Calming®, Lavender, StressAway™ in all my communities.

Occasionally, I had been fraught with doubt when listening to negative mind chatters. I had to turn off the mind if I wanted to move forward, which was full of fear and turn to my heart, which was full of faith, sunshine and guidance. I do this often by telling my mind to release negative thoughts; calling my spirit to the forefront; and practicing a breathing technique I call, Light & Love Breathing, which allows me to return to a place of power and love.

LIGHT & LOVE BREATH

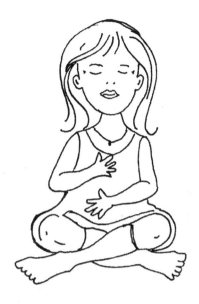

By placing one hand on your heart
and one hand on your solar plex
(just above the navel).
We connect with our powerful LIGHT
balancing it with our powerful LOVE.

This simple method will allow us to be who we are now in time and space. It is here where we will be able to listen to our own presence. When we are quiet, we will hear what we want and where we are going. First practice being who you are now. Feel it. Be with it. Love it. Gunilla Noris tells us, *Within each of us, there is a silence – a silence as vast as the universe. And when we experience that silence, we remember who we are.*

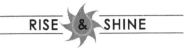

When you feel confidant of who you are, you can move into the question of what do you want? Do not ask others but listen to your Self. Allow your hands to rest anywhere on the body, then breathe consciously through your nose and into your belly. What do you want? Be still. Listen. Know. When the answers come, be prepared to write them down.

Sometimes, the answers to where we are going may come first and we can work backwards to what we want. This process is different for everyone. It is necessary to acknowledge the mind chatter, be okay with it, and then let it go with grace and ease. I believe the journey is right in front of us if we can give the Self the energy, vitality, and attention it needs.

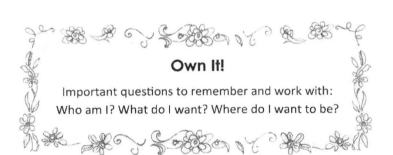

Own It!

Important questions to remember and work with:
Who am I? What do I want? Where do I want to be?

2

Voice It

Intentions, Friends & Family, & To Myself

DECLARING MY INTENTIONS TO THE WORLD AND MY DIVINE GUIDES

When I feel strongly about doing something, all I have to do is voice it to the world (or at least to my friends) and a series of dynamic motions go into effect to help make it happen. The Universe throws itself into alignment with the actuality of my bright ideas whenever I open my mouth and passionately express my plan. I believe our Spirit acknowledges who we are, what we want, and where we are going. Once we own and voice our intentions, we are on our way to making it happen.

I didn't get the CB handle 'Motor Mouth Mama' for nothing. I always had a big mouth. I couldn't move forward unless I was shouting my business from the top of a mountain. I let my voice be heard. Whenever I voiced it, I noticed more energy, vitality, and attention came to me through law of attraction.

I also noticed a deeper sense of ownership whenever I voiced my intentions, my plans. I became aware of the power in my declarations and affirmations to help me follow through with my ideas. When we declare our intention, we are owning it NOW and voicing it NOW. We are coming from a place of being in the present time. I repeat the following declarations:

- ≈ I love myself.
- ≈ I am living my passion.
- ≈ I own my story, my idea, and my expertise.
- ≈ I voice my intentions with confidence and joy.
- ≈ I am safe in the present.
- ≈ I am living life to the fullest and loving it.

Dad set a strong example on expressing intentions. He kept us up to date on his newest goals and intentions. Actually, he kept everybody apprised of his goals even the ones unrelated to business. Once when eating in a restaurant with the family, an acquaintance stopped at our table and said, "Hey, Hallie. What're you up to?" Dad answered the question with a detailed itinerary of our family weekend getaway. "About to hit the road after having breafkast (Dad talk) here with the family, heading up highway 70 straight through Kansas, stopping to park the rig for the night and then next morning, bright and early, heading for Denver to shop for some gear. Then jump back into the RV and heading for the mountains. Got reservations there at a pretty spot overlooking a valley where we'll call it a day and wake up the next morning and have a good breafkast (again Dad talk) and be on the slopes bright and early ready with our skis on." Then he grinned down at the family full of satisfaction over his plan, anticipating all the fun we were about to have, but I was already having fun just being with a dad who personified the word exuberance.

I learned to voice it from Dad. He voiced his personal plans, business plans, or family adventures or whatever activity he was currently involved in at the time. I loved listening to the excitement in his voice. I took on that excitement and sometimes even go overboard when telling my own family of all my intentions, but fortunately they have patience and smile at the genuine pleasure I feel whenever expressing what I am about to do.

When my boys were young, I always set the stage for the day, week, and sometimes the weekend. Now they are teenagers and have their own plans, which I enjoy hearing them express. I do notice they seem to possess an innate

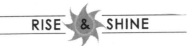

understanding of whenever their parents are happy going about their own daily business, life seems to go easier for them. They just no longer feel the urge to hear exactly what our business entails.

I have learned to voice my visions and desires to friends and people who actually care whether or not they come into fruition. My true people seemed to be the ones who understand my declarations and stay with me while I realize them with enthusiasm. The ones who show enthusiasm help to keep me excited about what I'm doing. They understand the power of what I see. I really do believe our Divine Guides are listening to what we have to say. My words go out into the Universe roll around for a while and then roll back to me in some kind of form.

Even though I had been using essential oils on my family and friends for years, I never really owned the idea of sharing my discovery with the world, but then when I owned it after going through the purification process in Ecuador and losing thirty pounds, I could tell something had shifted in me; I began educating others with breath, movement, and essential oils. When my family started noticing their benefits and making positive comments about my commitment to the well being of them and others, I just knew I had it going on.

So when I returned from Ecuador in 2009, it was a whole body transition, including weight loss, skin improvement, free

of pain, diet change, and a lifetime habit change. I put everything I had learned from my previous six years of experience
and added what I recently learned from my transformation
and decided it was time to take action by voicing my intention of sharing this knowledge with the world.

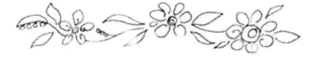

CALLING FRIENDS AND FAMILY

First though, I recognized the need to ask an expert on
marketing my own expertize. I turned to my husband George,
a successful sales man of seventeen years. He excitedly told
me to start by calling fifty people a day who I had helped with
essential oils. He said to tell them about my new passion for
owning the idea of sharing oils as a business, and then to tell
them I am here to answer any of their questions. I did exactly
what George told me to do. I called everyone even my family.
They loved the attention of my phone call. I could hear the
energy rise in their voices as I talked on about the benefits
of using essential oils and wanting to help them utilize these
beautiful oils for their own wellness needs. They, too, felt
lifted by the possibility of having more energy and vitality in
their lives.

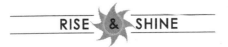

COMMUNICATION THROUGH EMAIL AND SOCIAL MEDIA

I then sent an email to everyone and invited them to a business builder meeting to join me in sharing and caring with essential oils. Twenty-two people gathered in the living room that night and eagerly listened to my contagious enthusiasm that came through my PowerPoint presentation. These twenty-two people became my Joyful Healing Oils Team, or as I call them JHOT mamas and men. It grew from the initial living room meeting of twenty-two to become a team of one hundred and fifty, and now just five years later, 2000 plus people work alongside my devotion of sharing essential oils with the world.

I love hearing people VOICE IT on social media. It is such a great venue to share our ownership of our new way of living by voicing it to our social media community. I was so proud of one of my friends recently who voiced his ownership in making diet changes to take gluten out of his life, apply his essential oils daily, breathe, and get moving with exercise to lose some weight and start living his life to the fullest with health and wellness as a plan. It is through this community that he will receive added energy, attention, and vitality to add to his own efforts and motivation. His community and the Universe will help make his declarations even stronger.

VOICING IT TO MYSELF

Whenever negative thoughts come in and grab ahold of my mind filling it with self-doubt, I practice one of the Native American traditions by drawing down the middle of a piece of paper, splitting it in half. On the left side, I write what I am releasing. I RELEASE... On the right side of the paper, I write what I want using the present tense. I AM... Then I read it out loud, applying Release™ and Forgiveness™ essential oils before reading the left column and Present Time™ essential oil while reading the right column, proclaiming it to the Universe. I wad it up and burn it outside in glass or metal. Then, I throw the ashes into the air to rejoin the earth. At exactly the moment the wind catches my ashes, I let go of all doubt and send out my new intentions by Voicing them to the world.

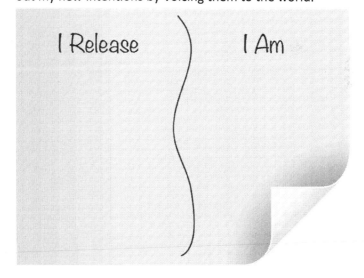

I Release | I Am

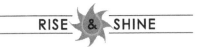

This practice can be applied to any negative thoughts, or feelings of fear, grief, despair that might arise from unexpected challenges. After releasing, we feel a sense of renewed vitality and can move forward with our intentions.

JOYFUL HEALING PRACTICE FOR VOICING IT

I practice voicing my affirmations by chanting and singing I AM, I AM, I AM to the rhythm of a Motown Marvin Gaye beat, swaying back and forth until my voice is so strong I can voice my intentions to the world. Sometimes, I use my favorite yoga version from the album *Flow* by Sat Kartar. I follow this practice with movement and breath, combining the following series:

CROWN BREATH

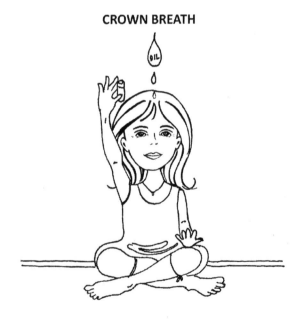

Sacred Frankincense Crown Breath – I drop 1-2 drops of Sacred Frankincense onto the crown of my head. I take my hands and rub through my hair where the oil dropped. Then I make a 'scent tent' in front of my nose and while belly breathing I inhale the beautiful aroma. As I exhale, I take my hands gently away from my face and place in prayer position. Inhaling essential oils helps us connect to the limbic system of the brain where emotions are stored. *All aromas have a potential emotional impact that can reach deep into the psyche, and both relax the mind and uplift the spirit.* – Linda Smith, author of *Healing Oils, Healing Hands.*

SCENT TENT

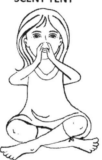

PRAYER TO HEART

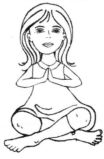

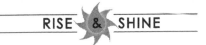

Reach for the Sunshine – Raise your arms like your grabbing the sun, inhale, make a fist and bring it to your heart, exhale while you say HAR three times, using a breathy sound. HAR means creative infinity, a name for God. Repeat several times. This is a great way to bring energy into the body.

REACH FOR THE SUNSHINE

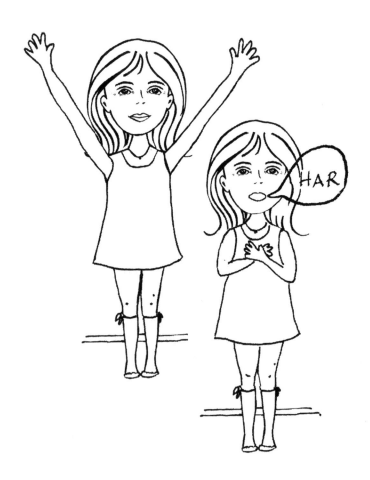

The Dynamic Forward Fold – Inhale when putting arms over your head and exhale while folding with a HAR. Be dynamic in this movement rising up and folding down. Repeat several times. Remember to make HAR a breathy sound. This is the mantra for prosperity.

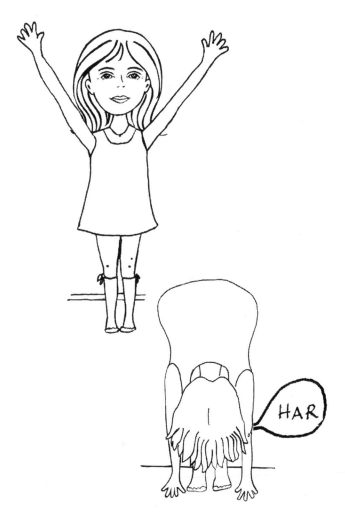

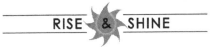

Throat Extension & Flexion - Sit in a comfortable position and lift your spine so your shoulders are straight and relaxed. Look straight ahead. Sometimes I apply the 1-3 drops of essential oils Eucalyptus radiata, Eucalyptus globulus, EndoFlex™ or Idaho Balsam Fir to my chest or my throat. As you inhale, look up while lifting your chin and closing your jaw. Pause. As you exhale, lower chin to chest. Come back to neutral, breathe normally, and repeat several times. This supports a release and opening of the throat to allow open communication.

THROAT EXTENSION

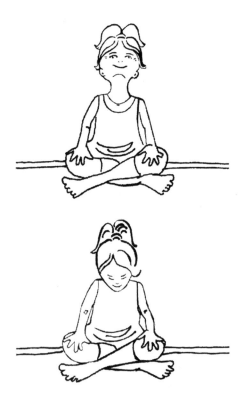

Affirmations & Declarations Practice – Sit in your most comfortable position, on the floor, in a chair, or on a blanket supporting your buns and be with your declarations and affirmations. I like to anoint my neck, heart, and feet or a combination of any with the essential oil Present Time™, Gathering™, Gratitude™, and/or Hope™. I find affirmations help me stay in a positive state. The following I AM statements are my daily practice:

AFFIRMATION AND DECLARATIONS

I am moving forward with grace and ease.

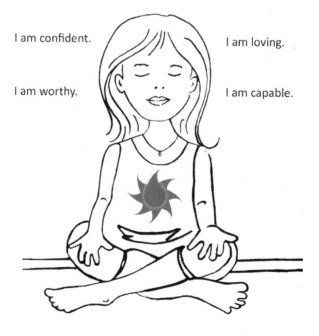

I am confident.

I am loving.

I am worthy.

I am capable.

Sit in your most comfortable position on the floor, in a chair or on a blanket.

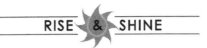
Allowing our voice to be heard and allowing ourselves to hear our own voice helps us get moving to our next step. The Universe hears us. Our friends and family hear us. We hear ourselves. Energy flows inward and outward to bring love (attention) to our intentions. Our energy heightens, which helps us write a plan with vitality. Now is the time.

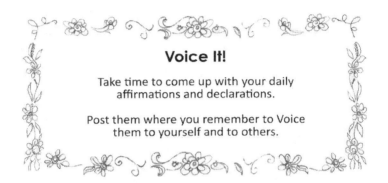

Voice It!

Take time to come up with your daily affirmations and declarations.

Post them where you remember to Voice them to yourself and to others.

3

Write It

Intention, Toleration List, & Radical Gratitude Chart

FAIL TO PLAN. PLAN TO FAIL

Dad bandied about this famous quote of Zig Ziglar's in our house like it was the Holy Grail. It rang loudly while I was growing up. My dad was big on writing out his plan and instilled this same philosophy in each one of his kids, myself included. Once when nine years old, I went to him with the simple request of taking our 26-foot Bow Cobalt boat across the lake to buy a gallon of milk and he said, "What's your plan?" I knew it had to be every last detail and include all of my action steps, so I replied, "First I need the money from you. Then, I have to lower the boat from the hoist to the water, untie it, put the key in the ignition and start the engine, making sure the boat

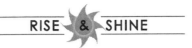

is in neutral first. Then, I put it in reverse and back out of the slip gracefully. Drive across the main channel up to Three Mile Cove to the Gas and Grocery. I pull up to the outer slip in low speed, taking it in and out of reverse to slow momentum and then let the dock hand help me tie it to the dock. I will go inside and buy a 2% gallon of milk from the clerk and use the same steps to return. Once I'm safely on the ground, I will hand you the milk and the change." (Since Ecuador, I discovered my body is happier without dairy.)

I knew Dad would let me do nearly anything I set my mind to so long as I had a plan. Later, I learned to write it down. My very first written plan was designed to get approval for my Peer Counseling Program in high school, which was a complete success, so from this I learned Dad was right and so was Zig Ziglar. The only downside came about by Dad's continued involvement in my need for a plan even into my thirties when he would call and ask what my financial plan was for starting a business, including making sure the number of hours I worked coincided with the amount of money I set as my goal. This annoyed me, and once in a while I would yank his chain by saying, "Well, Dad, just not feeling it, the need for a plan. Think I'll let things flow and see where it takes me. Maybe get a studio for yoga classes, and then get one of those Mini Coopers to use as a traveling office. You know the ones with the double back doors!" I could hear his chest constrict on the other end of the phone.

Of course, I had a plan; I was HIS daughter. He had hard-wired the program into my brain. Sometimes, I tried to fight it but when I discussed something I wanted to do with my business partner, invariably we would map the whole thing out and that would be the plan. The challenge for me was writing it down.

THE TOLERATION LIST

Once I owned and voiced what I was going to do, my mind would often spiral out of control with all the details. It felt like the many pieces that had to come together for the desired result could fragment at any second and spiral out of control. I began to feel paralyzed, numb, and spacy with the thought of everything there was to do and all I wanted to be. All I could think about was the puzzle coming together with a few missing pieces, the ones that fell out of my head while in the process of bringing my plan into a reality. That's when I remembered the concept of writing a Toleration List. I listed everything I had to do including the laundry, clean out the closet, clean the refrigerator, wash my car, set up my fall event on Facebook, update my website events, finish the day's email, and the million details needing to be done for the business, kids, home, and personal, which I put into categories. I called it a Toleration List because some of the stuff was just that – stuff I was tolerating but not doing.

Tolerations List

- laundry
- clean out closet
- clean the refridgerator
- wash the car
- set up my fall event on facebook
- update my website events
- finish day's email
-
-

I threw it all on paper just to get it out of my mind, clear some thought space so I could sort through everything and determine which ones were the legitimate action steps I needed to bring my plan to fruition. First though, I have to confess, whatever the mundane stuff was on my list like laundry, I did it just to get it out of the way or put a date next to it for doing later or write the name of who was going to do it for me! While writing out my list, I diffuse the oil of Clarity™ to support memory and mental alertness, which helps my mind clear and allows my brain the space it needs to activate my thoughts. Going for a meditative walk also helps clear my mind and brings about a sense of peace. I even read my favorite quote by Paulo Coelho when feeling overwhelmed. *There is one great truth on this planet; whoever you are, or whatever it is that you do, when you really want something, it's because that desire originated in the soul of the universe. It's your mission on earth.* I then follow this process with setting the big picture for my intentions.

RADICAL GRATITUDE CHART

Your vision will be become clear only when you look into your heart...who looks outside, dreams. Who looks inside, awakens.

~Carl Jung

A Vision Board is a very creative way of picturing your intentions. It's forward thinking and is also sometimes called a dream board or collage of what you want to bring to you. Vision Boards are both powerful and fun! The two words that I find most frightening are Dream and Goal. "Find your DREAM!" "Live your DREAM!" Well, some people may be able to easily find and live their one big dream, but for a few of us, there are many 'dreams'; it feels limiting to pick just one. I day dream all day long and sleep in dreamtime. This is powerful for me. Goal is scary and controlling to me, but it is a word that is difficult to replace.

I always created a Vision Board when setting about accomplishing a dream, but then when I felt challenged by an illness, I knew I could only be focused on a few things and needed to be grateful for all the good thing in my life.

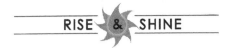

I started the Radical Gratitude Chart as another way to get moving with my core desires. I started saying out loud I am radically grateful for my oil business, my self-care, my legs that are giving me the message to slow down, and I'm radically grateful when my tired eyes remind me to spend less time on the computer. From this, I got the brainy idea that if I was challenged to get things done, then having a Radical Gratitude Chart could help me.

I love what Mary Jo Leddy said in her book *Radical Gratitude, We begin to recognize what we have rather than what we don't. We awaken to another way of being, another kind of economy, the great economy of grace in which each person is of infinite value and worth*. So after reading this, anything that made me angry, like my tired eyes, I turned into a sentence using radical gratitude to be grateful for what is challenging like the very word GOALS! The Radical Gratitude Chart makes them manageable, enjoyable, giving them a happy tone instead of feeling like a heavy burden. It allows me to get into what I'm working with rather than what I'm working toward. I have found the oil Transformation™ helpful in getting the energy to flow and allow change and growth.

My Radical Gratitude Chart usually lists 1 – 8 Projects I am gratefully working on during any given time. I apply one drop of the oil of Gratitude™ and write my core desires followed by a short phrase of what needs doing. Notice, I use the word 'doing'. I always used the word 'trying' but a good friend and teacher pointed out to me that if we are 'trying' then we are not 'doing'.

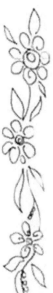

The next page is an example of one of my Radical Gratitude Charts. You can play with the blank one included.

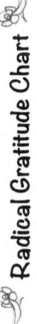

Radical Gratitude Chart

SELF-CARE Yoga, Breathing, Walking, Meditation, Cycling, Reiki, Personal Healing Appointments

BOOKS Rise & Shine: 6 Master Steps to Get Moving
Mom & Son Journey to Positive Health & Behavior

YOUNG LIVING Platinum to Diamond Increasing Income to $$$

YOGA CLASSES Teach X Amount of Classes with X Amount of Students

COACHING X Amount of Clients Per Month

U2IT Volunteer with Hospice - 3 Patients Per Week, Privates, Workshops

EVENTS Oil Wisdom Midwest ~ Fall 2014
Hormone Health ~ February 2015
Autism Awareness ~ April 2015

FAMILY CITY PLAN Look at Properties & Plan Budget

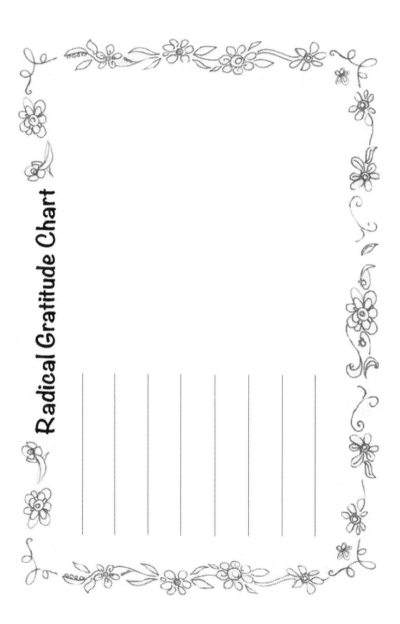

Radical Gratitude Chart

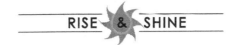
WORK BACKWARD FROM DESIRED END RESULT

I take my Vision Board and/or Radical Gratitude Chart and pick something from it; I look at my end result of where I want to be. In 2009-2010, I wanted to win a contest to be on the Young Living Mediterranean cruise, which required me to increase the size of my oil family. I worked backwards by setting goals each month on how many new oil family members I would need to accomplish my goal by the end of the contest. I worked diligently at this and by the end of the contest, I was number six in the world for increasing my oil family memberships.

This required me to schedule essential oil education afternoons and evenings every week either at the yoga studio, private homes, or in my own home where I educated people on wellness and how to utilize natural remedies for better health. The events were marked on my calendar along with the action steps to plan and prepare for these educational events. Even the simplest tasks, such as office store supplies with the list of goods needed would go on my calendar or reminder lists.

Sometimes forty people would come and sometimes it was only three. I showed the same level of enthusiasm no matter how many people were listening to what I had to say. My passion for wellness came through on how essential oils could be used to help support health and natural living.

When working backwards, we can see what is needed to accomplish any desire/goal that we list, put on our Radical Gratitude Chart, or have created using a Vision Board filled with pictures, affirmations, and handmade papers painted with footsteps or happy faces. We must look closely at the end result to know how to get there, what action steps to take, and how exactly everything fits into our calendars. It doesn't matter what we want the end result to be, whether crunching numbers for a dream house, writing a novel, losing weight, or building new relationships, we really do need to figure out what steps will get us there.

SET CALENDAR WITH DATES & DEADLINES

This requires me to get out my calendar and set the big dates for events, trainings, clients, and appointments that are important to accomplishing my desires/goals I have listed on my Radical Gratitude Chart, or in the old days whatever I put on my Vision Board. As an example for accomplishing my financial goals, if I want to make $1000 a month, I have to look at what it would take to make that amount. So once having determined how much I want to make, I now have to look at how much compensation I receive for each contact and once figuring out the math, I now know how many people I need to reach in order to make this happen. Once this is done, I can set the dates and their deadlines I need to put on

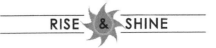
the calendar to insure this will happen. Now it's time for me to work my calendar by putting in the action steps to prepare for these dates and deadlines.

WRITE ACTION STEPS WITH DEADLINES

When I look at my Radical Gratitude Chart, I notice I am planning a Autism Awareness Event. **1.** I write on a separate sheet of paper the details and action steps of what I need to do along with my timeline. **2.** Get the speaker and set the date. **3.** Call the speaker and make sure her/his phone number is handy. Agree upon a date and mark on calendar. **4.** Once the date is set, I need to find a venue or physical site for that date. This requires much research, many phone calls, and voluminous email correspondence. **5.** Then I talk to my team of volunteers and get them excited about the speaker and promoting the upcoming event. This requires us to plan a meeting, which we then put on our calendar. **6.** At the meeting, we create a marketing plan to make the event a success. **7.** I set the budget based on how many expected ticket sales. (I use Excel to create a working budget.) **8.** I utilize an online service so I can keep track of ticket sales in order to set sales to what my venue will accommodate.

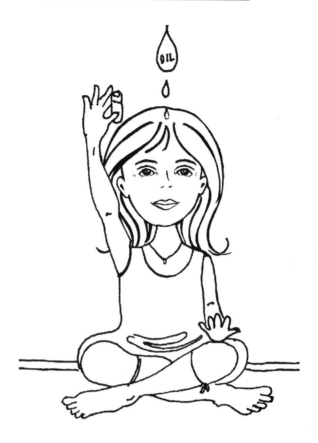

I like to use the oil Brain Power™ on the back of my neck and head for this process. It gives me clarity of thought, and helps me work well with others; it is uplifting and mentally energizing.

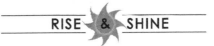

I also have a short yoga practice that gives me a boost of energy and keeps me zipping along.

BUNNY BREATH

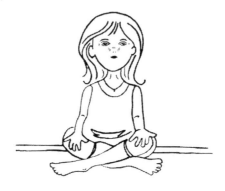

3 short inhalations through nose-like sniffing a flower
Long exhalation with mouth open and soft hah sound

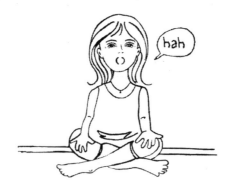

more oxygen & energy to the brain

CAT COW

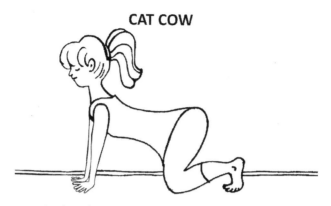

* On hands and knees
* Palms flat on floor, directly under shoulders
* Knees directly under hips
* Inhale concave spine looking up

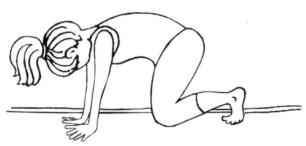

* Exhale,round spine looking through
  your legs like your're grabbing your cat tail
* Repeat 6x

moves and strengthens the spine

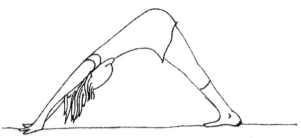

Downward Dog activates every muscle
in the body

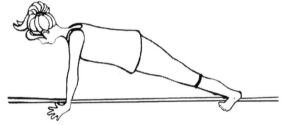

Incline Plane strengthens our core and power

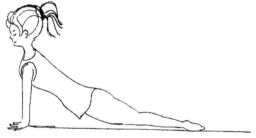

Upward Dog opens our heart center front & back

Upward Body Series - helps me sharpen my mind, come into focus, and strengthen my mind, body, and spirit through movement. As we are in Cat/Cow on all fours, let's tuck our toes under and lift our seats into Downward Dog. As we are here in Downward Dog, we feel our palms, flat into the earth as our arms extend allowing our armpits to lengthen and our shoulders to feel open. Our head is in between our arms with our ears in line with our arms. Our naval is lifted in and up taking out any exaggerated arch in the spine. Our seat lifts with the tale bone rising, yet sharpening slightly downward. Our feet are hip width apart. Our legs are extremely active lifting our kneecaps upward allowing our heels to come back to the floor any amount. After 15 years of yoga, my hamstrings and calves still will not allow my heels to touch the floor. It's all good.

Then we move into **Incline Plane** by bringing our seat down to allow our bodies to come into one line. We are lengthened so our hands are under our shoulders as we allow our shoulders to be in their sockets and our palms flat on the earth. The legs are active and lengthening through our heels. Our naval is strong in this pose as every muscle in the body is active. Breathe here and feel your strength and long body like a lizard on a rock. If stressed you can do this pose the YogaKids® way and look one direction and inhale, stick out your tongue, exhale and let out some sound! Repeat that on the other side. It feels good!

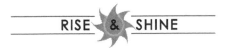

Next we move into **Upward Dog** as we slide our body forward through our hands at the same time as flipping our feet so the weight is on the tops of our feet now. Our upper body is lifted with straight arms lengthening through our side body. Our legs are active off of the ground allowing the muscles in the legs to activate. Our tailbone is lengthening towards our feet. If any of these postures are too much, we can skip them and always go into resting Child's pose. At this point, I apply or diffuse the oil of Surrender™ to support me in letting go the control I may desire in this process and I 'surrender' to Divine timing and order as I have set my Intentions, my steps, and my calendar into motion. Now I get moving with grace and ease.

CHILD'S POSE

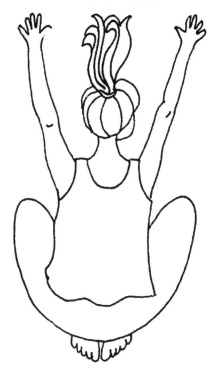

RESTING POSE

* Knees apart, toes together
* Extend arms out
* Extend spine
* Forehead to the earth
* Seat to the feet
* Rest and Breathe

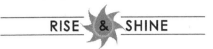

I believe the action steps are the most important pieces to the plan and can easily get overlooked. Sometimes, I write them in timeline fashion, and other times I work the steps on my calendar. Often these steps don't have specific times of day allotted to them, but I manage to work them into my day. This allows me to have time to do all my projects, including scheduling clients and personal appointments.

When I don't plan out my action steps, I feel overwhelmed and then want to retreat and do nothing. I find keeping up with my action steps gives a wonderful feeling of organization and freedom to shift and change and still know it will all get done in my own timing with the Universal energy working with me. I am a real fan of online calendars as a tool for helping me color code, move, and shift things without feeling like I'm just messing about. I get a great sense of freedom and breadth of vision when using online scheduling.

Once I have it all planned on paper or computer documents, I am free in both mind and body to work it! Just saying that makes me feel a sense of satisfaction like ahhhhhhh! After this process, it becomes about living day-to-day, balancing the tasks at hand, knowing that plan is my best friend. The plan is alive and always shifting and changing, but the intentions are set, the action steps are in motion, and now I am ready to GET MOVIN! And so are YOU!!

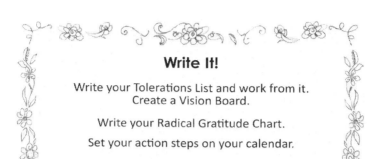

Write It!

Write your Tolerations List and work from it.
Create a Vision Board.

Write your Radical Gratitude Chart.

Set your action steps on your calendar.

4

Share It

Gathering Your Team, On Leadership, & Strength in Numbers

GATHERING YOUR TEAM

Dad never noticed being a real Mover in his industry but saw himself as just a guy with a plan gathering his team to help bring his vision into a reality. When the company became successful, he told us kids his business belonged to his entire family of employees and wouldn't be passed down from one generation to the next. With that in mind, he created the Employee Stock Ownership Plan for his company, which allowed the employees to be vested in the company. This gave real meaning to the word Ownership for his work family. Being generous by nature, Dad simply couldn't conceive of it being any other way. He was not motivated by greed but

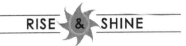
by helping people grow and become independent leaders while still keeping a sense of family and teamwork within the company. I watched Dad be a father to other people. When he saw potential, he wanted to help and he did!

Either I inherited this ability or learned it by his example. I notice I am compelled to have my yoga classes feel a sense of community and my oil members be one big oil-happy family. This exhilarates me, makes me feel like I am fulfilling my purpose in life.

I realized a long time ago, when putting a team together to help with my special needs child, how important it is to work with practitioners and doctors who are highly skilled in their area of expertise. I have always said, 'I know what I know and I don't know what I don't know'. I believe it takes a team to help us achieve almost anything worthwhile.

When I put my oil team together, I looked for people who wanted to go out in the world to share and care together. I did this by drawing from my own tribe, and that's what I tell my team to do, reach out to the people in front of them who are willing to give and receive, growing a business together, yet work independently. I also believe team building; growing and sharing together, have to come from a place of love in order to be authentic. Otherwise, the intention is motivated by greed. The concept of greed is not in my nature. It doesn't feel good to me. The only way I was able to build a team was by infusing it with energy, attention, and vitality, coming from a place of love. Then, I got busy helping my team become educators and leaders. Anointing with Gathering™ essential oil is also helpful in bringing people together on a physical, emotional, and spiritual level.

ON LEADERSHIP

I follow the motivational speaker Darren Hardy. He says it so well in the following statements posted on his website: *The leaders who will succeed going forward will be those who can build leadership in others. Leadership is no longer about getting others to follow you, but building leadership in everyone around you. You do this by developing the mindset and emotional intelligence (self-awareness, self-confidence and self-management) and skill sets (communications, time management, networking and team-building) so everyone can lead themselves in this constantly changing environment, thus leading you and the organization in the direction of your greater goals.* **It comes down to this:** *The winning leaders of the future will be those who can develop leaders out of everyone in their organizations the fastest.*

This amuses me when I remember Dad began practicing this philosophy during his barbershop days over fifty years ago. Even to this day, when we go out in his boat together, he lets me take the wheel but I can feel him suppressing his

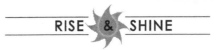

need to keep teaching me, although at this point in my life, I really don't need Dad to steer my course. I tell him he taught me well when I was nine years old.

I knew from the very beginning of starting my own business that there is strength in numbers. I wanted to build confidence in my team by increasing their knowledge about the benefits and use of oils for health and wellness. I encouraged everyone to become a product of the product so they could feel the benefits of using oils and talk to others by drawing from their own experience and conveying that experience with passion.

I mean, we're not selling Fuller brushes here. We are sharing health and wellness. The world expands a little when one person becomes well and full of vitality and aliveness. I love what Wayne Dyer says when talking about oils. *I believe what you are doing (with Young Living Essential Oils) is altering and shifting the consciousness of our planet!* That statement places importance on what I am doing with my life. I am basically on this planet to serve. I want to instill the largesse of this worldview in my team members.

I tell my team: BELIEVE IN WHO YOU ARE! They laugh at me like I'm their cheerleader, but I like to make what we're doing together fun, make it doable. During this process, I teach my team members not to overextend themselves either financially or with their time. I don't want them to think they have to spend a lot to make a lot in their business. It's necessary for them to learn to say no to events and opportunities that will not advance their plans. The word no becomes more powerful than the word yes. I teach them how to assess which activities are high payoff and which are low payoff activities. I find saying no takes a lot of confidence. Whenever I tell my team 'BELIEVE IN WHO YOU ARE', it helps to build their confidence, which in turn helps them to say no and even know when to say no.

I have found holding monthly meetings to share successes, knowledge, and comradery to be the most important element in building both a team spirit and leadership skills. Now, they all have their own teams and are successful leaders, holding their own meetings.

We often use the oil of Abundance™ to support magnetic energy and create the law of attraction through the magnetic field around us, which puts out a frequency charge of prosperity and abundance. I begin or end meetings by using a guided meditation.

The following is called The Circle of Awareness Meditation. Any oil of choice can be inhaled or dropped on your crown to bring about the desired result while practicing this meditation of awareness. I begin by saying: 'as we stand here, let's ground our feet, bringing our hands down to our sides and shaking our hands. Observe how your feel right now. As we stand here,

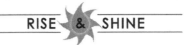
feel the energy go to the feet all the way into the earth. Feel the energy of the Divine within and all around us. To begin, let's spread love throughout the circle, repeating after me:

CIRCLE OF AWARENESS MEDITATION

There is Love above me.
There is Love below me.

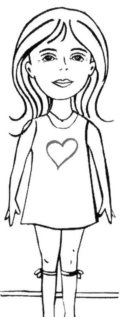

There is Love
in front of me.

There is Love
behind me.

There is Love
to the right
of me.

There is Love
to the left
of me.

There is Love within me.
There is Love all around me.

As we pass this essential oil around the circle, take a gentle inhalation of its scent. What is your first impression? (pause) Does it remind you of anything? (pause) Let's turn our attention to our breath as we breathe in this aroma. (pause) Now let's bring our attention to our body – where do we FEEL this oil going into our body? (pause) Notice how our body is receiving the aroma and molecules of this essential oil. (pause) Notice how our mind is receiving the essential oil. Let's feel it speak to us. Feel it move through us. Feel it help us. Feel it love us. (pause) Let's turn our attention to our breath as we breathe in these essential oils?

Can you name how the oil is making you feel? Can you sense some of the qualities and joyful healing this plant may offer you? (pause) Call on the powerful Plant world to bathe your body with wellness. Be direct and ask the oil to travel where you want it to go and ask it to give you what you want! (pause) Now bring your attention back to your breath and notice the essential oil perceiving you. Ask he/her if he/she has anything to share with you? Does he/she have a message for you? Now just listen. (pause) The plants and trees speak through their vibrational energy. You can feel and hear them speak if you listen from the wisdom of your heart. The essential oil is a living, pulsating being of great intelligence.

As we stand here together, let us Be in gratitude for the infinite generosity of the plant and tree kingdom. Let us Be in thanksgiving for Mother Earth and her enormous beauty,

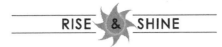

power, and joyful healing properties. Let us Be in gratitude for our Young Living Essential Oil Farms that support us with luscious plant and tree life to share through essential oils to the world. Let us express gratitude in our hearts.

Notice any shifts that have occurred in your mind, in your emotions, in your body? Notice this Circle of Awareness we have formed together and individually within ourselves.

Let's open our eyes and just Be for a moment. (pause) Begin to be aware and feel the rhythm of our breath. Feel the harmony in our soul. Feel the grace and ease in our body. Enjoy peace with the plants. Let's place our hands, one on top of the other, over our heart center. Repeat after me:

I am love.

I love myself.

I love others as much as I love myself'.

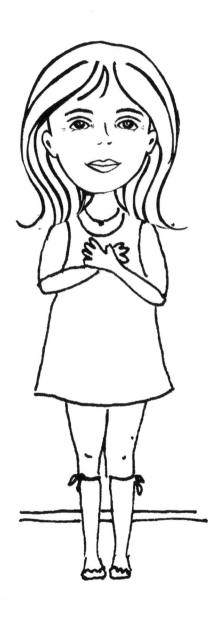

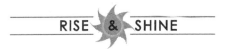
STRENGTH IN NUMBERS

I believe there is strength in numbers. This idea first came to me when both teaching and practicing yoga. I felt the vibrational energy of the group coming together, which added strength in our postures, our confidence, unifying the mind, body, and spirit connection. When I was alone doing handstands, I felt wobbly and weak but when in class, I felt strong and confident when the group was stronger than my individual energy. A group brings a WE BELIEVE sort of feeling that we get when others are standing by with encouragement and confidence.

The first time I went upside down, I had an emotional release and cried in class. It was challenging to stop crying. I could feel the fear leaving my body, the kind of fear that had been stored in my body for years. I wasn't the type of girl who hung from the monkey bars. Nope, too scary for me. The sense of being out of control and not grounded challenged me. I played football and basketball after school with a bunch of boys without the emotional song and dance problems; I never even feared being tackled by one of the boys. However, when it came to hanging upside down, I felt out of control and began to shake with dread. I realized that day my yoga mates were what grounded me when I went into my first handstand with confidence, even with the big sob fest afterwards. They supported me and allowed me to be my authentic self without judgment. I practice this same loving kindness in my yoga class and with my team and encourage it in others when they go out into the world for the first time to share their passion.

While making my own plans, I thought about how I could bring others into my plans to help all of us grow in our own strengths as well as together. I not only thought about building my own team, I always thought about how I could use what I learned along the way to help others build their team.

Now when studying my events and how to implement the work necessary to make them happen, I not only include my team mates but anyone else who wants to learn and share. This includes other organizations, other oils teams, which are considered competitors by most, but not me because I am motivated not by greed but by love. I feel there is enough energy, attention, and vitality to offer all people. I believe our passions will shine through when we work with integrity to support those who want to join us in elevating a common goal. There really is strength in numbers when we come together with people of like-minded values and desires. We are able to attract more energy and allow it to be manifested in all good ways by the Universe.

When sharing, I use oils like Motivation™ to help overcome fear and procrastination and take action in my life. Envision™, too, is a powerful support for balancing the

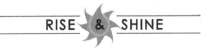
emotions in order to move forward with faith in the future in achieving dreams and goals. Magnify Your Purpose™ helps to support and uplift our emotional body, which in turn may help us overcome negative emotions and such self-defeating behaviors as procrastination and self-pity. It also may help us deal with feelings of abandonment, rejection, and betrayal. I find Highest Potential™ useful when wanting to empower myself; this blend may also be uplifting and inspiring while bringing about peace and stability. Needless to say, I don't use them all at once but instinctively know which ones will enhance my commitment to sharing at any particular time. My husband uses one of these oils after shaving in the morning to get his day off to a good start.

Everything I have to say about Sharing It applies to almost any goal or desire a person may hold dear to their heart. A wedding event, a birthday party, a new career can be a beautiful experience of teamwork when you bring others along for your journey, to share your most cherished times in a life that you can look back on and say it was lived in abundance.

The rhythm of the body, the melody of the mind, and
the harmony of the soul create the symphony of life.
- B.K.S. Iyengar

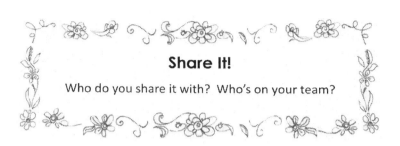

Share It!

Who do you share it with? Who's on your team?

5

Live It

Connect with Community, Experiment, & Walk the Talk

CONNECT WITH COMMUNITY

One of my favorite poems *Song of Myself* comes from Walt Whitman's book <u>Leaves of Grass</u>.

I celebrate myself, I sing myself,

And what I assume, you shall assume,

For every atom belonging to me as good belongs to you.

It's very important for me not to compare myself to others but instead celebrate myself. That's what 'living it' really means, enjoying every moment of the day and the celebration of each act no matter whether it is a task or a morning ritual to start the day. When we celebrate ourselves, we stay on task with our own work. We are able to work with our Radical Gratitude chart and stay on the journey we are walking. If I begin to compare myself to others, my desires get clouded and confused by the picture of others and what they are doing. It is important for me to sit and breathe in my own space daily, to practice on my yoga mat, and to share with people the gifts of natural living.

This is why I enjoy my morning ritual of waking up and getting ready to celebrate the day. I consider my Rise and Shine practice a way of celebrating myself. I believe when we live within our essence by Living IT, it becomes part of our day. I think this comes from living with purpose and abundance; the simple tasks become important to enjoy in and of themselves. They all go to together to give our lives a constant sense of the spirit residing within us. Living with wellness, purpose, and abundance is part of the Young Living mission. This falls in line with my natural way of being, the way I have always led my life as learned from my upbringing in a dynamic family atmosphere where business was life and life was business. Everything I do is not a business; it's a lifestyle. I tell this to my team, my audiences, and to my husband George.

Connecting with community comes naturally to me; I feel community is all around me. I love talking to strangers and sharing with them even if it's just a smile. I can become quite excited by it, but others who are with me are often embarrassed by my demonstrative nature. Once when sitting at the gate waiting to board a plane flying from London to the United States, I noticed a woman having difficulty breathing. People walked past her and boarded the plane like she wasn't struggling to breathe right in our midst. She kept frantically searching in her bag for something to ease the coughing. I walked over to her and asked if I could be of help. She shook her head yes.

I immediately went into my 'oil mode' and pulled out a bottle of Raven™ Essential Oil Blend. I have to qualify here that inhaling an essential oil is not always the best way to share essential oils with people who are struggling to breathe, but this situation seemed like an emergency and required immediate attention. Not to sound like a total woo woo, but I consulted my guides first and then did exactly as they said, which was hold the oil under her nose. Then I asked if I could apply some to her chest and again she shook her head yes. She began to breathe easier and after applying it to her chest, she took a deep breath and smiled. She hugged me and thanked me repeatedly. I gave her the bottle of oil to help her through the flight. Not only was she grateful but so was the flight attendant.

My husband George stood by watching in awe that his wife was brave enough to help a stranger. Previously, he had only seen me share oils with family members and friends. I think the work I do with others became real to George that day.

This is how I live it and how I connect with community. The world is my community. At the end of the flight, I bumped into the asthmatic lady. She told me she had a wonderful trip and went on to say her husband was a chiropractor in Chicago and would want to learn about oils. She asked for my card and became an oil lady herself. It felt like a pay it forward moment. We still keep in touch.

I believe 'living it' can apply to every person's way of being if they want to embrace what it is they have already owned, voiced, written, and shared, which then becomes the purpose of your life.

There are so many ways to keep in touch with community: social media allows us a vast electronic connection complete with images, personal, and professional updates; phone calls, Face Time, or Skype allows us to chatter endlessly across great distances; but the strongest connection is made in person where you can touch, see, and feel the person sitting next to you, and in my case, you can even smell the botanic essence of my daily oils.

Marcella Vonn Harting introduced me to Gary Chapman's book, *The 5 Love Languages*, which I use to help me optimize communicating by learning each of my team member's style and needs. I discovered through reading his book people feel connected in different ways including: words of affirmation (praise), acts of service, receiving gifts, quality time, and physical touch.

I have my clan and clients take the test for the 5 love languages, so I know their style and what they need. One friend needs constant praise and positively beams when I tell her she looks fabulous in her new shoes. Another one flashes a happy smile when I give her some small gift like the latest health food bar Young Living has put out. Another one likes it when I anoint oil on her tired shoulders, especially when she's in so much pain it's hard for her to string a few words together to form a complete sentence.

I encourage my clients and team members to take the time to connect with people in each of their preferred love language. It doesn't require giving everyone a test, but it does require being aware of what makes a person feel good. As a side note, figuring out your spouse's preferred love language goes a long way toward creating a harmonious household.

EXPERIMENT

While Dad may have laid the groundwork for the importance of organizing my life and having a plan, my mom was always my most enthusiastic supporter. When I suffered from various life challenges, she encouraged me to find alternative practitioners who could help me heal naturally without the use of allopathic drugs. She championed my yoga studies, oil travels and certifications, energy work certifications and practice, and all the other avenues I explored when coming up with 'a plan' to joyfully heal my own ailments and then took what I learned to help others. Embracing the holistic community rather than staying narrowly focused on traditional medicine was unusual for someone in her generation, but she has always been a person of spirit, faith, and strong intuition.

My friends have pointed out to me numerous times how Mom has the ability to give out love without expecting anything back. I appreciate this about her but also truly appreciate that she is still an ardent supporter of everything I do today. I think that's where I get the confidence to continue experimenting with various healing techniques. She was my first experiment allowing me to anoint her with oils to help support her in a grief from the passing of my grandma.

A major component of living it is experimenting. Recently, my son sprained his ankle while scoring three touchdowns.

He told me he only had three days to get back in playing shape for the next game. He asked me to use my oils to find something that would work in a short amount of time. We both grabbed the bottles and applied five different oils (Valor®, PanAway®, Wintergreen Lemongrass, and Peppermint) three times a day. By game time, he was in strong playing mode and ready to go onto the field where he scored another three touchdowns. (I also practiced energy work on his ankle but didn't tell him.)

Experimenting gives us that energy, attention, and vitality mentioned earlier and our intuition allows us to listen to the messages that come to us no matter what field we are in. We can have the courage to expand ourselves through experimenting, which ultimately helps us reach our larger goals. After all, Edison didn't invent the light bulb on the first try.

In the industry of holistic care without our testimonials, we don't always have proof that what we do works so we have to keep experimenting until something works. (Studies can be found on energy work and essential oils at pubmed. gov.) You can really feel it though when it does. In some cases, the experiment is helping someone learn how to feel. Living it is really about feeling but our fast paced society causes us to be constantly doing and doing. Teaching people to stop and Be has been a fun experiment. Then watching them Live as they Do and Be together is the best testimonial.

I think experimenting is essential in most fields or endeavors to come out with the best end result. I mean, how do we really know what we're doing now can't be improved upon, unless we're brave enough to try new things? Both my yoga practice and teaching classes are always an experiment. I feel the energy of that moment and go there.

My vet always laughed at me for believing my Cocker Spaniel's excellent health was due to living in an aromatherapy house, so I was greatly impressed by my vet's ability to experiment when hiring another vet in his clinic who uses acupuncture to help animals with their ailments. Even the new vet impressed me by the amount of courage it would take to needle the sick dog of a distraught dog parent who expected his dog to be treated with a pill. Never mind, sticking needles in certain points to get at the source of the problem. The world is now a better place because people are stepping out of their boxes and saying, 'Hey, let's try something new, different, and even radical'. The kicker to this story occurred when my old vet indicated an interest in listening to what I have to say about using oils and energy work to help animals.

Even a weight loss program requires a lot of trial and error with different diets and combos to find the plan that works for each individual. It took me a long time to find the diet and exercise combo that worked best for me. Living is going through these trials and errors to find what really works. Staying with the experiment long enough and with dedication is how we feel results.

I believe experimenting enlivens us, keeps us moving forward. I think this quote of Max Strom's sums up exactly what I've experienced with my willingness to try new ways of being. *Remember, it doesn't matter how deep into a posture you go – what does matter is who you are when you get there.*

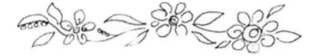

WALK THE TALK

Whenever I tell my team I'm a product of the product, it's my way of saying I don't just talk about how great something is without living it, which means I walk the talk. I believe we can only take people where we've been ourselves. I teach yoga sometimes several classes a week while also interweaving yoga throughout my day. Yoga isn't just about poses, it's also about awareness and attitude. I teach different breathing techniques, but I also spend time each day to sit and breathe consciously. While I may be in the business of sharing essential oils, I also use the same products to maintain my own health and vitality. I really believe in doing the work myself before I can even pretend to help others improve their overall wellbeing.

I also walk the talk in other ways. For instance, if a person needs a kind word, I listen. If a person needs to be relieved of pain, I assess what would help and offer a suggestion based on my experience. If they want to learn a yoga pose, I practice with them. I'm a very heart-centered person and am easily able to hear what a person needs when I'm with them or sometimes they just tell me, and I do whatever I can to help.

Walking the Talk also entails taking care of myself, which I do by practicing yoga, eating a pure diet, cardio workouts, and saying a blessing with gratitude when I stand before a mirror and see my face beaming back at me. I compare my body to a house in occasional need of repair and periodic rehab jobs. At these times, I utilize all the healing modalities I have learned and use them to heal myself. I am constantly searching for new ways of improving myself, my body, and giving peace to my spirit.

I find it necessary to check in on all aspects of life to help make sure I am living my authentic self. Through living it, we know who we are, what we want, and where we are going. When in Ecuador, Gary Young talked about practicing the **4 Questions to Living a Healthy Life**:

1. Daily devotion or relationship with God or Higher Power.
2. Attitude/passion for life.
3. Dreams for our life, goals, or desires. What do we want?
4. Our purpose that honors 1, 2, & 3.

So by asking these four questions, we have to take a look at our life and ask: why do I have this relationship with God? Why do I have this passion and this particular attitude toward life? Why do I have these dreams and desires? When we answer these questions, we are seeing the purpose for who we are, what we want, and where we want to go.

I have asked myself these questions so many times that they have become a part of me. I have them on my mirror as a gentle reminder of my purpose and to help me stay on the path I have set for myself in taking care of me, educating others, and sharing and caring for others. I have always felt that I am in the hands of God. I felt this when a small child standing by the creek and watching the water ripple over the pebbles, the sun shine and drop in rays on all the pretty wild flowers growing up the side of the creek bank, and when looking up and seeing all the fluffy clouds moving overhead.

My passion should be obvious by now. I Care!!! I Share!!! Being of service to others gives me an opportunity to say thank you God. And that is my purpose for being here in this world. My desire is inspiring love and healing through breath, movement, and natural living. I want to do this while feeling fulfilled and balanced in all aspects of my life.

The closest thing to the heart of God is restoring people.
When you take time to restore the broken, you pour the
healing oil on their wounds, encouraging them, wiping away
their tears, and letting them know there are new beginnings.

- Joel Osteen

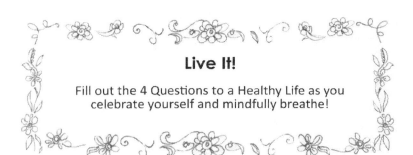

Live It!

Fill out the 4 Questions to a Healthy Life as you
celebrate yourself and mindfully breathe!

6

Love it

Authentic Self, Giving and Receiving, & Live What You Love and Love What You Live

This above all:
To thine own self be true,
And it must follow, As the night the day,
Thou canst not then be false to any man.
-Shakespeare, Hamlet

ATHENTIC SELF

I think of being authentic as being real. In my case, what you see is what you get. I operate in this world without façade. While this may make me vulnerable to negativity, I am the happiest just being me! Even though I learned a lot from my parents, I often didn't listen to them. I listened to my true self. They laugh about it now and say, "There was just no changing hard-headed Pam. She is who she is!" Whenever they say this, I smile, mostly because it's true, and it also reminds me that even when a child, I knew enough to operate from my real self.

I often wonder why I rarely hear people say someone is being authentic and usually when I do hear someone say this about another person, it's with awe in their voice. I could wrangle over this philosophical thought for several pages and it would always boil down to the same thing. Love can only come from the heart of a person who acts from their true nature, their authentic self. I have also observed when we come from this place, it is easier to inspire others with what we have to contribute to the world. I must have known this when a child, otherwise, I would have matured into someone I no longer recognized as being the original me. Frankly, I'd rather be me and happy than be someone else's version of myself. Yes, definitely, and I have also noticed I tend to surround myself with people of similar mind.

As mentioned, I tell my yoga classes, "We transform the body and the mind to meet the soul." When we calm our mind and become aware of our body, we are able to Be with ourselves, loving ourselves. I love myself is a strong declaration. When we love ourselves, we are able to love others. The Golden Rule says, 'Love your neighbor as you would yourself'. When I was a child, I took in the Golden Rule, understood it immediately. Later, I taught it in children's Mass at my church.

Really, I've been told I'm a preacher at heart. Even, my own Priest called me Priestess. Of course, my own family finds this all hysterically amusing. I try not to take myself too seriously, but there is a deep understanding of love that guides me.

We often describe ourselves by what we do when someone wants to know more about us. We say I'm the mother of three boys, a sales clerk, pediatrician, an author, or an oil lady. Who we are is not what we do; it's much deeper than that. We are a mixture of adjectives that express our true nature: kind, daring, creative, funny, positive, loving, loyal, honest, genuine, fearless, generous, and/or original. The list is endless. These words help us to express who we are. Why not use the adjectives to say who we are rather than say what we do when someone asks us? Again, in order to express this about ourselves, we have to love ourselves first. In loving ourselves, these qualities allow us to know what we want in our life.

When we know what we want and who we are then we can easily map out our radical gratitude chart, which will take us to where we want to be. I help this process along by using the essential oil blends Highest Potential™ and Into the Future™. Highest Potential™ supports me in elevating my mind as I gather my love and energy to achieve my own

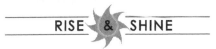

highest potential. Into the Future™ supports me in letting go of any past experiences and helps support me to get moving with vision, excitement, and vitality.

Loving what we are doing is the final Master Step. The other five steps helped us get to the place where we feel blessed in our own space and blessed by the Universe around us. As Joe Osteen says, So *we can wear our blessings well*. Now is the time to love what you are doing, shout it from the roof tops, and share the smile that's inside your authentic self with others.

GIVING AND RECEIVING

Gracious acceptance is an art – an art which most never bother to cultivate. We think that we have to learn how to give, but we forget about accepting things, which can be much harder than giving….accepting another person's gift is allowing him to express his feelings for you.

Alexander McCall Smith,
Love Over Scotland

My husband and I became best friends in high school. I learned a lot about giving and receiving love at this young age while being in love with a man I knew was my soul mate. We listened to each other with rapt attention, actually hanging onto every word as though everything we expressed to each other held endless fascination. We also possessed a knowing-ness or intuition about each other, a comfort that touched our spirit. It all felt like a soul connection, which allowed us to be our authentic selves. We could say anything to each other and not worry about being judged or criticized for expressing a half-baked idea or a crazy monologue of thoughts turned into verbal rants and possibly even idiotic expressions to anyone else but not to each other. No, we definitely found each other to be the most interesting person in our young lives and had no doubt that would always be the case.

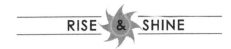

Here we are still married over twenty years feeling pretty much the same way. I do, however, notice George no longer hangs onto my every word but felt better after expressing this observation to a wise friend who told me that all husbands possess listening devices that can be turned off at will. He often calls my chatter 'nuggets of nonsense', which gets me laughing and reminds me I do occasionally think with my mouth. I have discovered that we don't really complete each other as much as we balance each other. The most important blessing that has been constant in our relationship is being able to understand that *when I love, I am loved*. This helps me move through my day giving freely to others without expectation and accepting what they have to give me with an appreciative smile.

In an effort to give back, I went to our Highland Flats Young Living Essential Oil farm in Idaho and helped plant five thousand Idaho Balsam fir trees in six days with twenty-two other people. So we gave to the earth by replenishing what we had received through harvesting trees that would have a short life span if left standing. There's a balance in giving and receiving when the earth nourishes the trees to help them grow. We harvest the trees in order to continue the cycle of giving through our Seed to Seal® process with Young Living Essential Oils. We then distill and bottle the essential oils to share with the world in hopes of supporting everyone's health and wellness.

I have always found the laws of nature worthy of observation. When a child, I could see there was a natural balance taking place in nature even though I might not have been learned enough to express it in words. Now, though, I have come to recognize the natural process of giving and receiving that takes place in nature can benefit our personal and professional life if nurtured in the same manner. I love the whole concept of giving and receiving as being inherent in all loving relationships. I mean really, it's the loving hand of God that causes the sun to shine on the trees. This thought makes me gleeful with happiness.

I teach a Giving and Receiving Breath, which can be done while standing or sitting. First you bend your elbows and place your hands on your shoulders. As you inhale, extend your arms out with palms up – giving. As you exhale, bring your hands back to your shoulders – receiving.

GIVING & RECEIVING BREATH

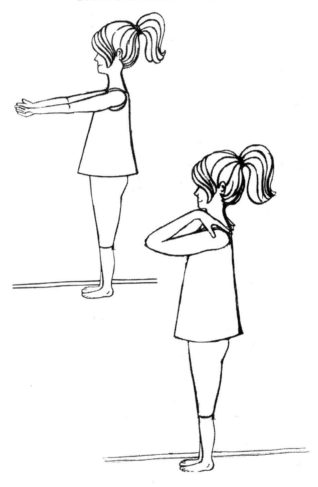

I see students practice this by over extending their arms as they give, which closes off their heart and shortens their breath. (This is a sign they are giving too much.) When they become aware and bring their shoulders back into their sockets, their heart opens and the breath fully flows, allowing them to receive breath and love as they give. In return, when they bring their hands back to their shoulders, they let go of a full exhale and feel completely balanced. This is a lesson I teach from my own personal movement practice that can be taken into our exchanges with others in the world.

I notice when I practice this movement before a professional meeting, I'm more open to giving my opinions and also receiving the opinions of others. I love this feeling!

~ Susan

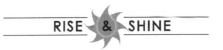
LIVE WHAT YOU LOVE AND LOVE WHAT YOU LIVE

Once we begin owning it, voicing it, writing it, sharing it, living it, we can now begin to love it with ease because we've put our Radical Gratitude chart into motion. When loving it, we experience joy from the process and turn it into a success. We can enjoy the path we are traveling without looking back and stay present while looking into the future. When we glance at the events on the calendar, we will be excited about the day's agenda while being present in that excitement. Loving it requires us to stay present so we've actually created a life full of joyful moments. A joyful moment occurs at the end of my day as I decompress by doing Leg Up the Wall, a joyful supine twist, and a self-hug.

LEGS UP WALL

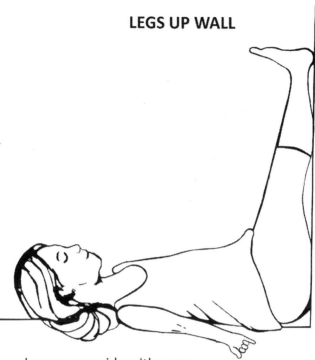

* Lay on your side with your knees hugged in and your buns as close to the wall as possible.
* Roll to your back and allow your legs to go up the wall.
* Buns are at the wall.
* Head lightly supported by a blanket if needed.
* Relax

Supports the circulatory system

JOYFUL SUPINE TWIST

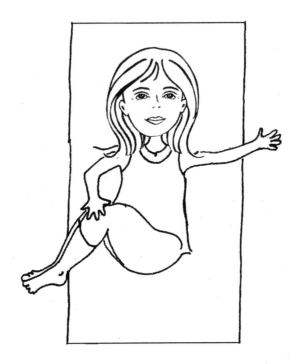

* Hug knees into chest
* Supine twist with knees to one side
* Switch knees to the other side
* Repeat several times with breath
  unwinds the day

SELF HUG

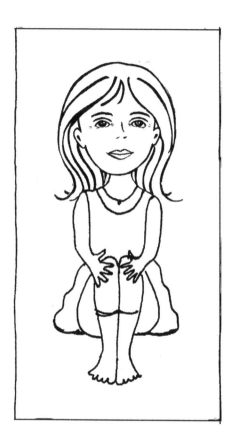

* Bring knees to chest in a hug
* Love yourself, rest and sleep

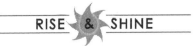
I also do volunteer work with Urban Zen Integrative Therapy. This program allows me to work with hospice patients, hospital patients, and anyone experiencing the PANIC-E model (pain, anxiety, nausea, insomnia, constipation, and exhaustion). It encompasses all the modalities I have practiced both personally and professionally over the years. This includes: Yoga therapy, subtle, restorative in-bed movements, body scan meditation, and breath awareness; essential oil therapy, inhalation method; nutrition; Reiki; and contemplative care.

I feel a real sense of loving it through helping patients who are hospital bound and don't have ready access to any of the holistic treatments. I also spend time with the caregiver family members. 'Bearing witness' is a large part of this time together where I listen without reaction. I have discovered my volunteer work keeps me balanced and is a blessing of giving and receiving.

Let the beauty of what you love be what you do.

– Rumi

When all of my years of working in these different practices come together to help someone, I feel blessed, blasted, and in a state of bliss! Life doesn't get any better than this for me. I love what I do and am humbled by the synchronicity and love of the Universal Power. I live in a wacky, joyful world of wellness and vitality. I hope you will join me!!!

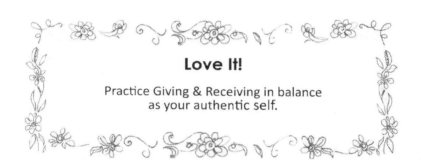

Love It!

Practice Giving & Receiving in balance
as your authentic self.

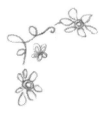

Own It!

Voice It!

Write It!

Share It!

Live It!

Love It!

May the long time sun shine upon you,
All Love surround you,

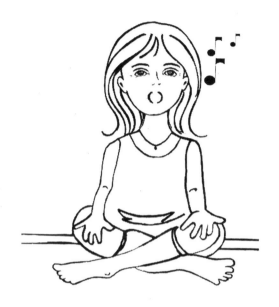

And the pure Light within you,
Guide your way on.

~Celtic Blessing

Sat nam!   Namaste!   God Bless!

I.

BREATHING APPENDIX

We take breathing for granted, because we all do it in order to live. But, there is more to breathing than we think. Breathing when practiced correctly can shift our mood, our energy, and our life! Through our breath, we can shift from sympathetic nervous system known as our 'fight or flight' mode to our parasympathetic nervous system known as our 'rest and digest' mode. As Americans, we often exist in the sympathetic, stressed-out, always on the go-mode like a hamster stuck in a turning wheel. If we stay in this sympathetic mode for long periods of time, we lose our energy and vitality and give our attention unnecessarily to extraneous detail. Learning tools to gracefully help us out of the sympathetic into the parasympathetic of calmness is golden for our body in allowing it to rest, relax, and re-cooperate. Belly Breathing & 3 Part Breathing are wonderful tools that I use to help this happen.

BELLY BREATHING

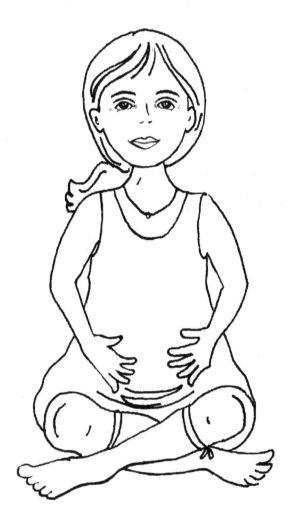

Belly Breathing, also known as a complete yogic breath, is when you inhale fully through the nose allowing your relaxed stomach to expand like an inflated balloon. You then exhale through your nose allowing the stomach to deflate and relax towards the spine. This action requires you to contract your stomach muscles until the diaphragm expands and presses upward into the thoracic cavity under the ribs. Don't think about it too much, just practice. Continue breathing until you have established a natural rhythm. Notice your belly will rise with inhale and fall with the exhale.

I like to put my fingers on my belly if I am sitting to feel the belly move. If I am lying down, a weighted object like a rolled blanket or a small pillow is nice to help me feel the rise and fall. This may be opposite to how we are currently breathing, but it is the way our babies breathe when entering this world. When we are about 3 – 4 years of age, we lose this natural rhythm due to taking on stress or 'fight or flight' behaviors. Now try and practice being a relaxed baby and begin to belly breathe.

When enjoying this rhythmic belly breathing, practice 3 Part Breath by:

1. Inhale first, concentrating on filling the belly and the lower lungs. **2.** Continue to inhale filling the middle lungs while feeling the rib cage expanding. **3.** Then inhale all the way into the upper lungs until feeling the collarbones

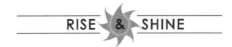

expand. As you exhale, first deflate your upper lungs, then your middle lungs, and then deflate the abdomen. Breath will be steady and rhythmic, like a wave rising and flowing in, and then flowing out again.

The objective of these exercises is to establish a new breath pattern of deep, full, even breaths. If practiced, these breathing techniques can help shift us out of stress (sympathetic) to relaxation (parasympathic) within minutes. Practice.

BREATHING TECHNIQUES PRACTICED IN THE 6 MASTER STEPS:

II.

YOGA APPENDIX

Yoga is the study of balance, and balance is the aim of all living creatures: it is our home.

~Rolf Gates

Yoga means union. In yoga, we work to unify the body, the mind, and the spirit to come into a harmonious state of being. For the body, mind, and spirit to be integrated, emotion, action, and intelligence must be in balance. The Yogis formulated a way to achieve and maintain this balance through the three main Yoga structures - movement, breathing, and meditation.

In Yoga, the body is treated with care and respect for it is the primary instrument in man's work and growth. Yoga movement supports all the systems of the body. By designing physical poses and breathing techniques that develop awareness of our body, Yoga helps us focus and relieves us from our everyday stress.

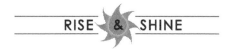

There are still a lot of misconceptions about Yoga being a religion. Yoga is not a religion. It is an art, philosophy, and practice for us to find spirituality. In fact, Yoga is practiced by a lot of people from different religions.

(This was co-written with Stacey Vann.)

Yoga helped me to become aware and *through awareness, WE transform the body and the mind to meet the soul.*
~Pamela Hunter

As you practice the postures in this book or any other yoga, please listen to your body and breath. If the breath becomes restricted as you move, listen and adjust allowing your breath to be your guide. Establishing a daily practice for your needs can be challenging. Reach out to an authentic yoga teacher to help you. With technology of today, there are many ways you can find help. You may want to visit, www.yogaalliance.org to find a teacher or studio near you.

YOGA MOVEMENT PRACTICED IN THE 6 MASTER STEPS:

Point & Flex p. 21
Ankle circles p. 22
Self hug p. 23
Roll out of bed p. 25
Tarzan tap p. 25
Extended mountain pose p. 26
Standing twists p. 27
Neck circles p. 28
Rag doll p. 29
Rise & shine p. 30
Reach for the sunshine p. 48
Dynamic forward fold p. 49
Throat extention & flexion p. 50
Affirmations and declarations p. 51
Cat/Cow p. 67
Upper body movement p. 68
Child's pose p. 71
Circle of awareness meditation p. 80
Legs up the wall p. 111
Joyful supine twist p. 112
Self hug p. 113

Urban Zen Integrative Therapy Program was inspired by Donna Karan, Rodney Yee, and Colleen Saidman Yee. You can find more information about this program at www.urbanzen.org.

III.

OILY APPENDIX

Young Living is not a perfume business. We are in the business of wellness. It is not how good the smell of the essential oils are, but how effective the oils are in helping a person's body to heal itself.
~ D. Gary Young

Essential oils are a huge part of my life! I feel blessed to know them and love them! In this section of the book, I share my relationship with Young Living Essential Oils: my many favorites, how they make me feel, how I use them, and perhaps how my family uses them. Let's have some fun lovin' oils!

In this book, I share my two favorite ways of using oils. When I anoint myself with essential oils, I am using the topical application method. This method can be applied 'neat' meaning without a carrier oil (a fatty oil such as olive, almond, coconut, jojoba, etc.) or with a carrier oil on the area of need, or on the bottoms of the feet. My favorite places to anoint others and myself are on the bottoms of my feet, around my naval, on my heart, on the back of my neck, and/or the crown of my head. I enjoy essential oils in my baths with Epsom salts as an emulsifier to mix the oils into the water.

The inhalation method is another effective way of using essential oils. I like to carry peppermint with me but do not necessarily want to smell like a candy cane all day. So I use the inhalation method with peppermint often, as well as other oils, depending on my mood. Diffusing essential oils is a powerful way to inhale them. Letting the tiny oil molecules float into your environment and enter into your olfac-

SCENT TENT

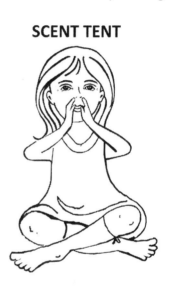

tory receptors and your limbic system is joyfully healing! When I start up my kitchen diffuser in the mornings, it helps me to Rise & Shine and get moving!

Now, let's get to know the oils in my arsenal! Please understand these are my favorites, how I use them, and what they do for me. ***These statements have not been evaluated by the Food and Drug Administration. They are not intended to diagnose, treat, cure, or prevent any disease.***

Pamela's Oil Arsenal
Physical

Drinking Buddies
Lemon
Peppermint
Lavender
Slique Essence™
Orange
Spearmint
Ocotea

Outside of Eyes
Lavender
Juniper
Copalba
Helicrysum™
Frankincense

Lymph Flow
Cypress
Aromalife™
Lemon

Earth Mamas
Valor©
Grounding™
Patchouli
Cedarwood

Sleepy ZZZ
Palo Santo
RutaVala™
Ylang Ylang

Breathing Pals
Raven™
RC™
Eucalyptus globulus
Rosemary

Breast Awareness
Idaho Balsam Fir
Frankincense

Colon Ease
DiGize™
AromaEase™
Lemongrass
Peppermint
Spearmint

Bug Defense
Thieves™
Purification™
ImmuPower™
Eucalyptus Blue

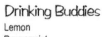

These statements have not been evaluated by the Food and Drug Administration.
This product is not intended to diagnose, treat, cure, or prevent any disease.
Refer to your Essential Oil Desk Reference

PAMELA'S PHYSICAL OIL ARSENAL

DRINKING BUDDIES:

Lemon – I put 3- 6 drops in a glass of water before I go to bed so it is ready for me to drink first thing in the morning. I was taught that if we drink water before anything else in the morning, it hydrates our organs before they start to work. Nice! The lemon is said to help support the balance of alkaline vs. acidity in the body.

Peppermint – I put ONE drop in a large GLASS pitcher of water in my kitchen and pour from that pitcher into my own GLASS. One drop of peppermint essential oil is equal to 28 cups of peppermint tea – so ultra strong. This is minty fresh and soothing to the digestive system and it cools the body inside and out.

Lavender – One of my favorite drinks to make in the summer is Lavender Lemonade. Fresh squeezed lemons, water, ice, a bit of Stevia or agave for sweetness and just a few drops of Young Living's lavender. YUMMY!

Slique Essence™ - This blend of Grapefruit, Tangerine, Spearmint, Lemon, Ocotea, and Stevia tastes fabulous! Some days I drop it in my glass of water and other days, I swipe the side of the bottle with my finger and then swipe the oil inside my lip and gums for a refresh. Now, I am not telling you how

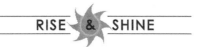
to use your oils, but I enjoy the taste and benefits of this oil tremendously. It may support healthy weight-management goals and support our digestive systems; this means a lot in my life!

Orange – I love to add a few drops of orange essential oil to my NingXia Red shot in the morning. What is NingXia Red? Check it out on my website: www.joyfulhealingoils.com.

Spearmint – We love spearmint for its minty, fresh taste; it soothes the movement of acid flowing up that needs to move out instead. A drop in water, similar to peppermint, but more soothing for that up and down flow of uncomfy digestive juices.

Ocotea – This single oil has a spicy, fresh scent and a taste similar to cinnamon but more subtle. I like this oil for its support to our digestive systems and blood sugar fluctuations. Just a drop will do it for me.

OUTSIDE OF EYES:

I like to put roller ball caps on all of these bottles and use these bottles around my eyes. I make one circle around the OUTSIDE of my eye socket, layering them on one after the other - **Lavender, Juniper, Copaiba, Helichrysum, Frankincense**. If you want to know why I use these oils, I suggest looking up their properties in the Essential Oil Desk Reference. I have had some major eye challenges, and I consulted with Gary Young who never told me to put essential oils in my eyes, therefore, I will never put oils in my eyes on purpose.

LYMPH FLOW:

Cypress – One of my all time favorites; it supports the circulatory system and lymphatic system with grace. I place 3-6 drops on the bottoms of my feet and up my legs before going Legs Up the Wall to release swelling in my feet, ankles, and legs.

AromaLife™ - Another favorite of mine supports the cardiovascular system. Think about its name. I add this oil blend of Sesame Seed Oil, Cypress, Marjoram, Ylang Ylang, and Helichrysum to my Epsom salts baths. One cup of salt to 5-7 drops of oil for my bath. When you add Epsom salts to your bath, you are absorbing the mineral Magnesium and the essential oils you add to it.

Lemon – Fresh and soothing to my digestive system first thing in the morning and throughout the day is lemon essential oil! As mentioned earlier, it is one of my 'drinking buddies' but I also like to diffuse it throughout my office and my home to lighten the mood while it soothes and helps my inner fluids flow!

AromaSeiz™ - When I feel like my body is tense with occasional spasms and needs to let go, I like to add this oil of Basil, Marjoram, Lavender, Peppermint, and Cypress to my Epsom salts bath, too. It is soothing to my muscular body.

EARTH MAMAS:

Valor® - This blend of Fractionated Coconut oil, Spruce, Rosewood, Frankincense, and Blue Tansy is the signature blend of Young Living Essential Oils, in my opinion. I personally use it every morning and throughout the day many times. I use the roll on to put it on my cervical spine and into the LC notch at the edge of the hairline. It is my grounding and centering oil that helps me protect myself from outside energies and influences. It helps me to focus and concentrate on just being me.

Grounding™ - This blend of White Fir, Spruce, Ylang Ylang, Pine, and Cedarwood are many of my favorite single oils all put together! The tree oils shine with the balance of ylang ylang and helps me ground in the moment while coming into reality. This is my 'put my feet on the earth, buckle down and do it' oil!

Patchouli —I love how this thick oil feels on the skin when I apply a few drops topically, but I really love how it helps me lower fluid retention and inflammation. I apply a few drops to my lower belly and bottoms of my feet and then enjoy a scent tent!

Cedarwood – Often people put Earth Mama oils on their feet, but I like it on my head! I like to anoint my head with a few drops on my crown; it feels so yummy sweet and is also great for hair re-growth! With all the health challenges I have experienced, this is a win/win!

Sleepy ZZZ:

Palo Santo – I have a special relationship with this oil, which we call a brother to Frankincense. I enjoyed the Palo Santo forests during my trips to our farm in Ecuador. The Palo Santo is rich there. We distil the tree bark lying on the earth. George loves his Palo Santo; it supports his sleep without any waking or snoring. He applies so much that I can just lie next to him and breathe to experience the same effect. He applies a few drops on his temples and back of his neck like he is making the sign of the cross before bed! So great! He couples this with RutaVala™ for Sleepy zzzzzzzzzzz's!

RutaVaLa™ - This is a proprietary blend of *Ruta graveolens,* Lavender and Valerian. It is soothing to stressed nerves and supports relaxations to the mind and spirit; it is a favorite in our busy household. The scent grows on you and smells quite nice when layered with other oils such as Palo Santo. This is the second oil my husband applies at night while he's blessing himself.

Ylang Ylang - I prefer the sweetness, balance, and beauty of Ylang Ylang. It is ultra-special to me because I was in Ecuador when it was first planted, then when we were able to pick it years later and distill it. A beautiful yellow flower with wonderful relaxing properties and tenderness! This is the oil I smell in Peace & Calming™. I like to spritz or diffuse it in my room at night and other times in the day when I need my mind to rest.

BREATHING PALS:

Raven™ - This blend of Ravintsara, Lemon, Wintergreen, Peppermint, and Eucalyptus radiata was mentioned in the book as my very first oil ever used for my son and me. The story shared in the text says it all! It will always be our favorite oil for supporting our respiratory systems. I often apply just a few drops for comfort when needed, just because I love the smell.

RC™ - This blend of Myrtle, Eucalyptus globulus, Marjoram, Pine, Eucalyptus citriodora, Lavender, Cypress, Eucalytpus radiata, Spruce, and Peppermint was the second oil we ever used in our household. RC™ was the sidekick to Raven™ for both of my boys. But for my son Charlie, RC™ won as his favorite from age 5-7 years; it helped him clear the gunk he was constantly swallowing. Just a few drops to his chest nightly was joyfully healing!

Eucalyptus globulus – Of all the eucalyptus oils, this one is my preference for its pure eucalyptus scent. It is what you'd expect to smell when smelling eucalyptus with its fresh, opening, and inviting aroma to our airways. Diffusing and applying topically are good ways to use this oil effectively.

Rosemary – I like to put a drop of rosemary in my neti pot! Talk about a WOW!

BREAST AWARENESS:

I feel it is extremely important to bless ourselves with our own touch. Our breasts are a part of our body needing some attention. I anoint my breasts with two oils, **Idaho Balsam Fir and Frankincense** (any of the frankincense family members), by layering on a few drops of each and massaging it in. This is supportive to the lymphatic system and helps us to love our selves physically and emotionally.

COLON EASE:

DiGize™ - This blend of Tarragon, Ginger, Peppermint, Juniper, Fennel, Anise, Patchouli, and Lemongrass is soothing to our digestive systems; it helps allow whatever needs to go, to go! We all use this in the Hunter house for those occasional belly rumbles, motion sickness from carnival rides, and just to make sure things are moving! Sometimes inhaling it is enough. We inhale, diffuse, apply, and once in a while, it will get into my mouth.

AromaEase™ - A new gentle blend of Peppermint, Spearmint, Ginger, Cardamom, and Fennel. This has become my personal favorite to soothe my belly when bloated, gassy, and noisy – yes, it happens to most of us! Just a few drops to the lower belly is so soothing!

Lemongrass – I love to eat lemongrass, and I also love the smell of the oil! Just a few drops is soothing to my digestive

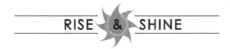

system. Sometimes, I like to add it to coconut oil and massage it into my entire abdomen. It feels nice.

Peppermint - As I mentioned in the 'Drinking Buddies' section, it is nice to add it to water or tea, but when I am nauseated, I put a drop under my nose and let it soothe my occasional tummy upsets, quickly!

Spearmint – If or when I eat late at night or have popcorn, a couple drops of spearmint on my middle chest is soothing to those angry digestive juices that need to calm down and settle.

BUG DEFENSE:

Thieves® - There is just so much to say about this oil blend of Clove, Lemon, Cinnamon Bark, Eucalyptus radiata, and Rosemary. We put it on our feet everyday before school when the kids were little. Now, we use all of the products in this product line in our home. It is the product that is in our lives the most and used in so many different ways – hand soap, toothpaste, mouthwash, floss, household cleaner, hand sanitizer, and diffuser.

Purification™ - I mix 3–6 drops of this oil blend of Citronella, Lemongrass, Rosemary, Melaleuca alternafolia, Lavandin, and Myrtle in my natural laundry detergent daily! We also diffuse tons of it!

ImmuPower™ - This blend is our go to oil for when we feel something is coming to get us! 1-3 drops on the bottoms of our feet helps us feel stronger. Hyssop, Mountain Savory, Cistus, Ravintsara, Frankincense, Oregano, Clove, Cumin, and Idaho Tansy make a powerful supportive blend for our immune systems. *When my boys were little, I would apply 1-3 drops of **ImmuPower™** to the bottoms of their feet and put them in the bathtub to soak for a bit. Then I would apply 1-3 drops of Frankincense up their spine and put them to bed. They would sleep and wake up feeling stronger and better.*

Eucalyptus Blue™ - This is our Ecuadorian eucalyptus. It has a very strong scent and very strong properties. When I feel like I need support in a major way, I reach for Ecualyptus Blue and apply 1-3 drops or diffuse.

Pamela's Oil Arsenal
Emotional

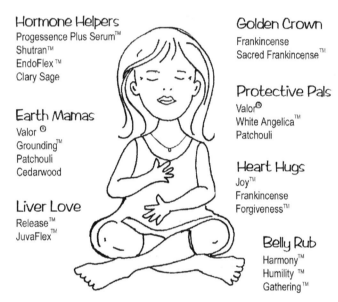

Hormone Helpers
Progessence Plus Serum™
Shutran™
EndoFlex™
Clary Sage

Earth Mamas
Valor ®
Grounding™
Patchouli
Cedarwood

Liver Love
Release™
JuvaFlex™

Golden Crown
Frankincense
Sacred Frankincense™

Protective Pals
Valor®
White Angelica™
Patchouli

Heart Hugs
Joy™
Frankincense
Forgiveness™

Belly Rub
Harmony™
Humility ™
Gathering™

Creative Clearing™
Idaho Blue Spruce

Hanky Panky
Idaho Balsam Fir

Playful day
Orange
Inner Child ™
Present Time ™

Nervous Nellie
Idaho Balsam Fir
Frankeincsnse
Basil
Marjoram
Aroma Seiz ™
Common Sense ™

These statements have not been evaluated by the Food and Drug Administration.
This product is not intended to diagnose, treat, cure, or prevent any disease.
Refer to your Essential Oil Desk Reference

PAMELA'S EMOTIONAL OIL ARSENAL

HORMONE HELPERS:

Progessence Plus Serum (PPS) – My progesterone is always low or non-existent. How do I know this? I do blood work with Dr. Dan Purser. He helps create this product for YLEO and guides me medically. I drop a couple drops of PPS (see the ingredients in the Essential Oil Desk Reference) on my inner elbows and then take some from there and rub on the left side of my neck in the front. It smells great, making it an enjoyable nightly routine. It keeps me happy and sleepy.

Shutran™ - A favorite of my husband's morning routine as aftershave with a few other oils. This blend of Idaho Blue Spruce, Ocotea, Hinoki, Ylang Ylang, Coriander, Davana, Cedarwood, Lemon, and Lavender gives George a skip in his step and a happy bliss for the day and night.

EndoFlex™ - This combination of Sesame Seed Oil, Spearmint, Sage, Geranium, Myrtle, German Chamomile, and Nutmeg support the Endocrine System. I apply a few drops to my soft organs around my mid-section and in the front of my neck as support when I feel this system needs it. Plus, it smells great and feels warm!

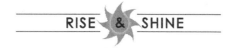

GOLDEN CROWN:

Frankincense – Boswellia carteri is my personal favorite of the frankincense oils; it was the first one I ever used. It helped me tremendously with my moods and feeling happy, healthy, and holy. I still to this day, drop 1-2 drops on the crown of my head and let it anoint me with its golden properties of joyful healing. I traveled with Young Living along the Frankincense Trail in Egypt and Jordan in 2010 and was in Gary Young's *ONE GIFT* movie with my frankincense testimonial. One of my favorite memories – riding a camel in the middle of the desert in the sunshine dressed as an ancient Egyptian – classic.

Sacred Frankincense – Boswellia sacra is truly a gift to us. I interchange all of the frankincense oils and love every one of them. I call them the King of Oils!

Three Wise Men™ - A lovely anointing of Almond Oil, Sandalwood, Juniper, Frankincense, Spruce, and Myrrh to the crown of my head or third eye to go deeply into a meditation practice is a gift!

EARTH MAMAS: Listed earlier.

PROTECTION PALS:

Valor® - As mentioned earlier, I use it daily and throughout the day by dropping it on or rolling it on. It is my protection oil and also grounds me with the armor needed to Live and Love it!

White Angelica™ - This blend of Fractionated Coconut Oil, Myrrh, Bergamot, Sandalwood, Geranium, Ylang Ylang, Spruce, Rosewood, Coriander, Hyssop, Melissa, Rose, and Angelica is a grand protection! As I apply just 2 drops in the palm of my hand to rub gently across each shoulder, I feel the power of these oils shield me energetically from anything negative. I then rub the remainder in my hair so it can naturally diffuse throughout the day. The scent is beautiful and has been known to attract the opposite sex if this is what you desire.

Patchouli – Also mentioned earlier but as a protector; I apply 3 drops to the bottoms of my feet and up my legs to feel the sensation of walking strong and steady!

HEART HUGS:

Joy™ - It only takes a drop for me to feel its comfort; I apply this blend of Bergamot, Ylang Ylang, Geranium, Lemon, Coriander, Tangerine, Jasmine, Roman Chamomile, Palmarosa, and Rose to my heart or chest area – it's happiness in a bottle of beautiful aroma!

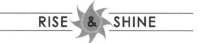

Frankincense – Any of the Young Living bottles applied to my heart or head gives me great relief and comfort knowing I am accepting a beautiful hug from our earth!

Forgiveness™ - We all have times when we need to forgive others and ourselves. This little bottle is a powerful yet gentle reminder to forgive; it comes in a blend of Sesame Seed Oil, Melissa, Geranium, Frankincense, Sandalwood, Coriander, Angelica, Lavender, Bergamot, Lemon, Ylang Ylang, Jasmine, Helichrysum, Roman Chamomile, Palmarosa, and Rose. As I place a few drops on my heart, chest, or naval, the scent enters in allowing me to take a breath of awareness and forgiveness. Wonderful!

LIVER LOVE:

Release™ - We all have a little anger stored in us some-where. Well, this oil blend of Ylang Ylang, Olive oil, Lavandin, Geranium, Sandalwood, and Blue Tansy gives me great comfort while letting go of stored emotions. I apply just a few drops right over my liver area. This oil is a powerful support to our emotional bodies!

JuvaFlex™ - This blend of Sesame Seed Oil, Fennel, Geranium, Rosemary, Roman Chamomile, Blue Tansy, and Helichrysum supports our liver and lymphatics. The scent is soothing and wonderful when I anoint my soft organs of the liver and kidneys with this supportive emotional oil blend.

BELLY RUB:

Harmony™ - In times when I am feeling my energy all over the place and outside my body, I know I need support to balance and clear. This blend of Sandalwood, Lavender, Ylang Ylang, Frankincense, Orange, Angelica, Geranium, Hyssop, Spanish Sage, Spruce, Coriander, Bergamot, Lemon, Jasmine, Roman Chamomile, Palmarosa, and Rose helps to restore my energy centers and brings about wellness. I use 1-3 drops around my naval and then enjoy a scent tent!

Humility™ - In joyfully healing myself through many health challenges, this oil is a wonderful gift of Fractionated Coconut Oil, Coriander, Ylang Ylang, Bergamot, Geranium, Melissa, Frankincense, Myrrh, Spikenard, Neroli, and Rose. With just a few drops around my naval center, I feel a stronger frequency and connection to God, Mother Earth, and myself.

Gathering™ - Support physically, emotionally, and spiritually, this oil blend of Lavender, Geranium, Galbanum, Frankincense, Sandalwood, Ylang Ylang, Spruce, Cinnamon Bark, and Rose, is felt when inhaling this beautiful feminine scent. When I feel the need for this blend, I put a drop on one hand, rub my hands together 3 times, then hold one hand at my naval area and one hand at my nose and breathe.

Forgiveness™ - As mentioned earlier in Heart Hugs, I also apply this blend around my naval as it support balance to our entire being.

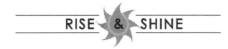

PLAYFUL DAY:

Orange – This clean, citrus scent is definitely playful; it brings me into my inner child mind. I love to diffuse it in the kitchen to freshen the house and my mind!

Inner Child™ - Scent stimulates memory responses. This oil blend of Orange, Tangerine, Ylang Ylang, Jasmine, Sandalwood, Lemongrass, Spruce, and Neroli supports me as I reconnect with my inner-self. I use this oil with my Light & Love Breathing to get back into my true self.

Present Time™ - Being in the moment is such a gift and often a challenge. This blend of Almond Oil, Neroli, Spruce, and Ylang Ylang supports the present moment. I put a drop on my thumb and place my thumb in my mouth touching the roof of my mouth. Then I suck my thumb for just a bit. Yes, it's playful, fun, and my mind becomes present.

CREATIVE CLEARING™:

Idaho Blue Spruce – When I feel the need to clear some old emotional patterns and refresh into my present affirmations, I use this special oil. There are specific points we place this oil to clear. But I also love the scent because it takes me back to our Idaho farms. Just a few inhalations of this oil is powerful!

HANKY PANKY:

Idaho Balsam Fir – Drip, drip, drop and let yourself and your partner explore!

NERVOUS NELLIES:

Idaho Balsam Fir – Another woodsy oil scent that supports my nervous system. When I apply 1-3 drops topically or diffuse, I feel supported when my 'nervous nellies' melts away.

Frankincense – I have mentioned the effects of this 'King of Oils' throughout because it has been my main support to my nervous system by helping me to come into my highest potential and walk strong. Just a few drops on my head or heart or a quick inhalation does wonders for my psyche!

Basil – I think of basil as a 'nerve tonic' because it is supportive to all of our nerve pathways. This is one I choose when I feel challenged in my joints and spine. I apply 1-3 drops topically for support and comfort.

Marjoram – An oil to support us during occasional times of tension is a great tool! For me, this is marjoram. When I have tension, it shows up in my back, shoulders, and joints. Just a few drops topically on those areas are so helpful to me.

AromaSeiz™ - My nervous system likes to be jumpy at times. To settle and relax my body, I put 3-5 drops of this blend of Basil, Marjoram, Lavender, Peppermint, and Cypress in my bath with Epsom salts. I do like to place a drop or two on location topically if that area needs extra help in settling.

Common Sense™ - A drop on the crown of my head of this blend of Frankincense, Ylang Ylang, Ocotea, Goldenrod, Ruta, Dorado Azul, and Lime is just enough for me to wake up to here and now thinking.

Pamela's Oil Arsenal
6 Master Step Oil

OWN IT

Believe,™ Valor®
Harmony,™ Joy™
White Angelica™
Frankincense
Idaho Balsm Fir
Helichrysum™
Thieves,™ Myrrh
Peace & Calming™
Lavender, Stress Away™
Raven,™ RC™

WRITE IT

Clarity™
Transformation™
Gratitude™
Brain Power™
Surrender™

LIVE IT

Valor ®
Pan Away®
Wintergreen
Lemongrass
Peppermint

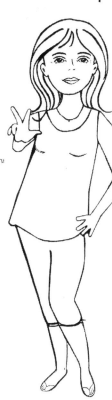

VOICE IT

Present Time™
Release™
Forgiveness™
Sacred Frankincense™
Eucalyptus radiata
Eucalyptus globulus
Endoflex™
Idaho Balsam Fir
Gathering™
Gratitude™
Hope™

SHARE IT

Abundance™
Gathering™
Motivation™
Envision™
Magnify Your Purpose™
Highest Potential™

LOVE IT

Highest Potential™
Intro the Future™
Lavender

These statements have not been evaluated by the Food and Drug Administration.
This poduct is not intended to diagnose, treat, cure, or prevent any disease.
Refer to your Essential Oil Desk Reference

PAMELA'S 6 MASTER STEPS OIL ARSENAL

OWN IT:

Believe™ p. 31

Valor® p. 31

Harmony™ p. 31

Joy™ p 31

White Angelica™ p 31

Frankincense p. 34, 35

Idaho Balsam Fir p. 34

Helichrysum™ p. 34

Thieves® p. 34, 35

Myrrh p. 35

Peace & Calming™ p. 36

Lavender p. 36

Stress Away™ p. 36

Raven™ p. 19, 91

RC™ p. 19

VOICE IT:

Present Time™ p. 45, 51

Release™ p. 45

Forgiveness™ p. 45

Sacred Frankincense™ p. 47

Eucalyptus radiata p. 50

Eucalyptus globulus p. 50

EndoFlex™ p. 50

Idaho Balsam Fir p. 50

Gathering™ p. 51

Gratitude™ p. 51

Hope™ p. 51

WRITE IT:
Clarity™ p. 56
Transformation™ p. 58
Gratitude™ p. 59
Brain Power™ p. 65
Surrender™ p. 70

SHARE IT:
Abundance™ p. 79
Gathering™ p. 77
Motivation™ p. 85
Envision™ p. 85
Magnify Your Purpose™ p. 86
Highest Potential™ p 86

LIVE IT:
Valor® p. 95
PanAway® p. 95
Wintergreen p. 95
Lemongrass p. 95
Peppermint p. 95

LOVE IT:
Highest Potential™ p. 103
Into the Future™ p. 103
Lavender – With the purity of Young Living's lavender, I call it the Queen of Oils! If I don't know what to do, I use lavender.

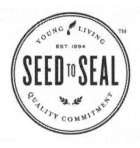

It is important to note that I share Young Living Essential Oils because I believe in our Seed to Seal® quality.
www.seedtoseal.com

I grew up with parents who were raised by farmers, and I hung out on my Grandparents farm growing up, which makes me a farm girl at heart. Our farms with Young Living Essential Oils are special to me, because we work together and Love It!

If you are inspired by this book and want to learn more about Young Living Essential Oils, the Joyful Healing Oils Team is here for you! We LOVE to educate! It is easy to find us at www.joyfulhealingoils.com. We would love to have you join our Wacky, Joyful World of Wellness. You can educate yourself with the Essential Oil Desk Reference by D. Gary Young. You can also learn from these websites and find more resources about Young Living Essential Oils.

www.youngliving.com
www.oil-testimonals.com
www.lifesciencepublishers.com
www.crowndiamondtools.com

You can also find us all over Social Media!

About the Author

Pamela Hunter's journey on the path to wellness has provided her with the opportunity to heal from her many health challenges throughout the years by being open to inspiration and shining forth with grace. She feels blessed by her friends and practitioners (both holistic and allopathic) who came into her life in Divine order at just the right time. Her path has guided her to learn and grow, living life to the fullest. Through these experiences, she knows how important it is to be consistent and practice self-care daily to stay in the best health possible. Living this journey with joy, laughter, and a positive attitude, inspired Pamela to write this book.

Pamela is Founder and Director of Joyful Healing overseeing 2000+ members; certified in several healing modalities: Clinical Aromatherapy using Therapeutic-Grade Essential Oils, Spiritual Healing, Reiki, and Reflexology; Registered Yoga Teacher with Yoga Alliance since 2005; Urban Zen Integrative Therapist; internationally known Integrative Nutrition and Health Coach; launched the Joyful Healing Oils Team in 2009; and was

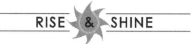

Awarded No. 6 in the world for recruiting new members to Young Living Essential Oils in 2010. Hunter writes a monthly column for *Be Healthy* section of the *Glancer Magazine*. She resides in Chicago area with her husband and two grown sons. She is at present traveling, speaking, writing, and still growing!

She has much to share and more books are coming.

Work with Pamela to be mentored through these 6 Master Steps to Get Moving and establish your own self-care to live and love it!

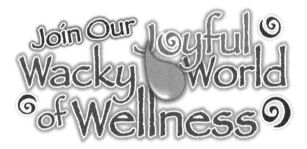

www.joyfulhealingoils.com

References

Chapman, Gary. *The Heart of the 5 Love Languages*. Chicago, IL: Northfield, 2007. Print.

Hardy, Darren. "WOW Beginnings (2 of 2)." *Darren Hardy, Publisher of SUCCESS Magazine |*. Darren Hardy, n.d. Web. 02 Dec. 2014.

Harting, Marcella Vonn. *The Harting Training System*. Phoenix, AZ: Yes No Maybe Publishging LLC, 2007. Print.

Higley, Connie, and Alan Higley. *Reference Guide for Essential Oils*. 2013 ed. Spanish Fork, UT: Abundant Health, 2013. Print.

"MODALITIES." *Urban Zen Integrative Therapy Program RSS*. Donna Karan, 2008. Web. 06 Dec. 2014.

Smith, Linda L. *Healing Oils, Healing Hands*. 2nd ed. Arvada, CO: HTSM, 2008. Print.

Whitman, Walt. *Leaves of Grass by Walt Whitman: The 1892 Edition*. New York, N.Y.: Bantam, 1983. Print.

Wenig, Marsha. *YogaKids: Educating the Whole Child through Yoga*. NY, NY: Stewart, Tabori, & Chang, 2003. Print.

Young, Gary. *Essential Oil Desk Reference*. 6th ed. N.p.: Life Science, 2014. Print.

Young Living | World Leader in Essential Oils | Young Living Essential Oils. Web. 02 Dec. 2014.

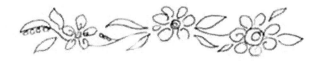

Notes

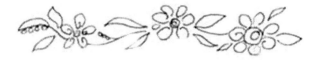

Notes

Made in the USA
Lexington, KY
04 September 2017